the SlimPreneur

the Slim**Preneur**

How To **LOSE** *Weight*
While You **Make** *Money*

JANET K. FISH

NEW YORK

the SlimPreneur
How To **LOSE** *Weight While You* **Make** *Money*

ISBN 978-1-61448-357-1 paperback
ISBN 978-1-61448-358-8 eBook
Library of Congress Control Number: 2012945259

Morgan James Publishing
The Entrepreneurial Publisher
5 Penn Plaza, 23rd Floor
New York City, New York 10001
(212) 655-5470 office • (516) 908-4496 fax
www.MorganJamesPublishing.com

Cover Design by:
Rachel Lopez
www.r2cdesign.com

Interior Design by:
Bonnie Bushman
bonnie@caboodlegraphics.com

In an effort to support local communities, raise awareness and funds, Morgan James Publishing donates a percentage of all book sales for the life of each book to Habitat for Humanity Peninsula and Greater Williamsburg.

Get involved today, visit
www.MorganJamesBuilds.com.

To my friends and family who have always given me unconditional support – you know who you are!

And to Michael, for always being there. "And we're still together."

Table of Contents

Foreword

by Loral Langemeier

"It's about time!" was my first thought when I read through the first few chapters of *The SlimPreneur*. In my many years of mentoring and coaching thousands of entrepreneurs, I've noticed a very distinct pattern in those that have mastered how to make money – they take care of themselves first!

Finding balance between your professional and personal life can pose a whole new challenge for the highly driven, and all too often, the sacrifice to "have it all" comes at the cost of our own health.

That is until now! Janet Fish is not only a very dear friend of mine, but also a fellow coach. She's helped hundreds of clients reach success and it's through this experience that she's been able to enter the mind of the entrepreneur and unearth the misconceptions about building a business while keeping a focus on weight loss, health and fitness.

As a single mom of two, owner of multiple businesses, speaker, author, trainer and entrepreneur, Janet and I have shared health and fitness strategies for years along with how to stay fit amidst the travel, family, managing employees and hectic schedules.

It's all too easy to get "caught up" in the day to day in your quest to be on top and believe it or not, many successful people put themselves last – telling themselves that they'll work hard, make a lot of money and take time for themselves when they reach the top.

The truth is that you need to be at your best to be your best, and finally there's a "How to" blueprint in *The SlimPreneur – How To Lose Weight While You Make Money*. Janet's delivery of simple and easy tips and techniques will show you how to have your health and company too!

Like my book, *Yes! Energy – The Equation to Do Less, Make More*, this book captures the power of how changing the way you think will change what you do and ultimately bring the positive and amazing results to the slim, fit and wealthy person you desire and deserve to be!

The Slimpreneur busts through the myths and misconceptions that weigh you down and provides that "missing link" on how to lead a healthy AND wealthy lifestyle – it's time to stop waiting for one to have the other!

Say "YES!" to your health and your future! Read this book, do what Janet says and share your success story!

—**Loral Langemeier**
"The Millionaire Maker" and five time NY Times Best-selling Author

Introduction

As more Americans aged 40 to 60 have been laid off, they are turning their attention to starting businesses of their own. New business startups averaged 565,000 a month in 2010. Further, more and more folks between the ages of 20 and 35 are turning away from traditional career paths, seeking to carve their own way with a business of their own.

What too many discover is that the path to a great career–independent of a large, established company–may gain them riches but it also wreaks havoc with their health. Weight gain settles on their hips and belly as they spend more time working on lean costs instead of lean eating, on mental stimulation instead of physical exercise, and on corporate fitness instead of personal fitness.

We are experiencing the worst recession and depression since the Great Depression of the 1930's. America has lost over 800,000 jobs, the majority of which will never return. People have lost their homes and their incomes and are asking the question, "Now what?"

As Americans come to terms with the likelihood that they won't find a company to go to work for, they face the inevitability that their options are government entitlement programs or creating their own means to support themselves. More and more people are joining the ranks of small business owners, seeking to start or grow their own businesses.

I started out to write a book about the unique challenges of starting a new business or successfully growing an existing business. As I interviewed current and aspiring entrepreneurs about what they thought were the keys to a successful business, something quite interesting kept coming up. While the focus was clearly on creating or growing a business, a large majority of the people I talked to also mentioned the desire to lose weight and improve their health and fitness. An alarming 80 percent or more of them said that after making money, losing weight and getting fit was their second most important goal. I certainly can relate to that, although I've been a successful entrepreneur for many years, I have always kept a keen focus on my health and fitness.

No one really understands the challenges of *not enough time* like the entrepreneur. When you work for a large company and have a *job*, you work your 8 hours and go home. When you're an entrepreneur you are the company, responsible for all divisions and responsibilities. Sure, you hire people to do many of the tasks, but ultimately the buck stops with you. For many the demands of the job leave little time left for taking care of **you**. Although exercise, healthy eating and fitness are a priority, it somehow gets moved to "I'll do it tomorrow," where tomorrow never comes.

In *The SlimPreneur - How to Lose Weight While You Make Money*, you'll learn the secrets successful entrepreneurs know, the better you take care of yourself, the more successful your business will be. I'll share the short cuts and strategies that ensure you meet your weight loss and fitness goals no matter how busy your schedule is. You'll learn to think like a healthy and wealthy entrepreneur and how those unique thought patterns make the difference between success and failure.

The better you take care of yourself, the more successful your business will be.

The SlimPreneur came into existence because, like many other entrepreneurs, I face unique challenges when trying to manage my business as well as my weight and fitness.

After quitting my W2 job many years ago I created a number of businesses, primarily in real estate, but my real passion has always been coaching other existing and aspiring entrepreneurs. I've been coaching wealth building since 2005 with a well-known organization that educates and creates millionaires. After coaching hundreds of clients, I came to the realization that a very large percentage of successful entrepreneurs struggle to balance the demands of their business with their desire to lose weight and be more fit. I can relate; I've been working to keep slim my whole life. Using my years of personal experience with weight loss and fitness, combined with what I've learned coaching hundreds of business professionals, I've created coaching programs that meet the specific needs of the entrepreneur and busy business professional. If the client does the work, he or she will see results. I've seen this in my business coaching and I've seen it in the fitness realm.

I wrote this book initially for me. To be quite honest, I thought I'd write a book about weight loss and make money. Now, I still do intend to make money with this book, but along the way I discovered something quite different emerging as my "Why." I'll talk at length about the concept of our "Why" in Chapter 2, but right now it's enough to say your "Why" is your *underlying* reason for doing anything you do—not the surface reason, but the deep-down inside, won't-stop-till-you-get-it-done reason.

I'll admit that I like money and I've been rather successful, but money doesn't drive me. I've always known that the main reason I coach is to give back. I've been quite blessed in my career with great skills that I've used to be successful and I've been fortunate enough to have made a lot of money. However, it was only during the process of writing this book that I came to realize that coaching—specifically coaching entrepreneurs and busy business professionals—was my gift and I had better start spreading it around. I believe it is our responsibility as adults inhabiting this planet to make a contribution and return to others some of what we have been blessed to receive. It's just good energy and for me it is exceptionally satisfying.

I've focused on entrepreneurs first because I am one, and second because entrepreneurs face unique challenges as they juggle growing their business, spending time with friends and family, all while trying to stay healthy and fit. Often we push health and fitness to the back burner, even though we know with certainty that healthy habits spill over into all other areas of our lives actually making us better at what we do, whatever we do.

> Often we push health and fitness to the back burner, even though we know with certainty that healthy habits spill over into all other areas of our lives actually making us better at what we do, whatever we do.

I wrote this book so that I could reach as many people as possible with a message of having it all. Fitness, health, wealth, everything you desire in your life is right there, if you claim it. The work is not always easy, but the rewards are worth it. I hope you find this book useful. If you do, share it. Give it to a friend who might benefit from it, or better yet, buy a copy and give it as a gift.

To get the most out of this book, complete the exercises that appear at the end of each chapter. The exercises compliment each other and will ultimately give you a good starting point for your weight loss and fitness plan. You can complete the exercises by writing in the book, or log onto http://www.slimpreneur.com/resources/ to download the exercise templates. Go download them now so you can build your weight loss and fitness plan as you work through each chapter. You'll find the exercise templates as well as many other useful and free resources on our website.

Don't be a stranger; we'd love to hear from you. Stop by our website at http://www.slimpreneur.com and share your journey. Our goal is to change people's lives, one day at a time. I hope you will join us.

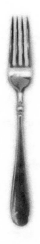

CHAPTER 1:

Current Weight Loss Strategies and Why They Don't Work

Not everything that is faced can be changed,
but nothing can be changed until it is faced.
—James Baldwin

With the obesity rates climbing higher and higher in this country, you don't have to go far to find people who want to lose weight. The realization that with weight loss comes greater self-esteem, self-confidence and increased energy has many folks making the commitment to some kind of weight loss program or solution.

Many people, when they find they have had enough, finally decide it's time to make that commitment to themselves. They choose a method or program, plan or diet (a word I abhor). Perhaps they follow a program suggested by one of their friends or colleagues. Maybe they've seen an ad on TV for a weight-loss solution and decide it's the one for them.

Negative Perceptions of the Marketplace

Regretfully there are plenty of people out there looking for a fast and painless solution that claims you can lose weight without changing your eating habits or adding exercise to your routine. I think we all know there are no silver bullets or magic pills, much as we'd like to believe the claims.

The other day I was at the gym on the elliptical machine, which in my gym also has a TV attached. I usually listen to my iPod, but I had run out of battery power so I found myself flipping through the channels. I came across an ad for a new weight loss product so I paused to see what they were selling. Research I like to call it. Lots of bikini clad women and buffed dudes showing their "amazing results." This product promises you can continue to eat all of your favorite foods and still lose weight. You just sprinkle the product on your food and you lose weight.

I was sufficiently intrigued by their claims that I came home and did a Google search on the product. I did some looking around and found that not only did the product not work as claimed, but their "30 Day Money Back Guarantee" was bogus. There were claims by many who had purchased the product that they had tried and tried but had been unsuccessful in getting their money returned.

> Any program, pill, potion or gadget that promises quick weight loss, or weight loss success with little or no effort, or any other claim that seems too good to be true, *is too good to be true.*

I don't mention the company name on purpose because I don't mean to single out any one company or product; I just use this as an example of all the weight loss scams that are out there. Any program, pill, potion or gadget that promises quick weight loss, or weight loss success with little or no effort, or any other claim that seems too good to be true, *is too good to be true.*

One of my biggest pet peeves is the use of celebrity spokespeople who endorse weight loss products. I don't include spokespeople like

Marie Osmond or Kirsty Alley who promote programs on which they have enjoyed success. They are only endorsing what has worked for them and I support that. It's the celebrities who endorse products for cash that I find the most offensive. These folks use their fame and notoriety to convince others that they can lose weight fast and easy, without significant change, and they get paid to do it.

Fad Diets and Cleanses

Fad diets and cleanses are also methods of weight loss that I caution against. I've tried a number of them and can't with good conscience recommend them. Fad diets aren't sustainable. They may work for a while—I've known many people who have lost weight this way—but I've known few who have kept the weight off. The good thing about fad diets (yes, there is one good thing about fad diets) is they are easy to follow. You are so limited in what you can eat that you have few options to get in trouble.

The bad things about fad diets are many. They are hard to maintain for any length of time; they don't teach you good eating habits; they have a horrible track record of maintaining weight loss; and most important of all, they can be dangerous to your health. Many of these fad diets recommend you only stay on them for limited periods of time. Why do you think that is? Because they can hurt you!

Cleanses are another category altogether and shouldn't be considered a weight loss strategy. I've done two extensive cleanses in my life. Both were 30 days in length. The first cleanse I did was primarily for weight loss. I was promised that I could lose lots of weight fast with their meal replacement products. I followed the instructions to the letter and lost 11 pounds in the 30 days. I was happy with the result, but quickly gained the weight back. However, the program had other side effects. The first two days I felt like I had the worst hangover ever—like I'd been hit by a truck. I was told that it was my body releasing all the toxins, which may be the case, but next time I think I'll pass. The other major side effect was a total lack of energy and strength. I've always been active and athletic but during the cleanse, I was restricted to eating so few calories that I couldn't even work out. That program is in the "never do again" category.

The purpose of my second cleanse was to release toxins from my major organs; it did not require me to severely restrict calories. Although I struggled with the taste of some of the products, I endured and made it through the 30 days with only a minimum of cheating. Hey, nobody's perfect.

Through those experiences and the research I've done, I don't believe in cleanses for weight loss. I don't think they work over the long term. I believe sustained weight loss comes from dedication, commitment, hard work, focus and support.

> Sustained weight loss comes from dedication, commitment, hard work, focus and support.

What's Your Excuse?

In my experience as a coach I have found some common complaints, excuses really, that come up again and again. As humans we love to tell ourselves things that just aren't true. "I don't have the time" is one of my favorites. I wish I had a dollar for every time one of my clients used the excuse that they don't have enough time. While it may seem like time is scarce, it's not really. You see, we all have the same amount of it. The difference is how we use our time and the way we prioritize our time. I believe that using time wisely can be a way to increase the effectiveness of our ability to manage our lives and what we want to accomplish in our lifetime.

I'll give you an example. A dear friend of mine is one of the top women on the speaker circuit and runs a successful multi-million dollar company. She is the busiest person I know. Her schedule would make most people fall right over. She travels extensively both domestically and overseas. She made nine trips to Australia last year. Yet she has unending energy. We were talking about that the other day as I was sharing with her some thoughts I wanted to include in this book. She said, "Janet, you know because you do it too, it's all about establishing a routine and sticking to it."

We both work out every day, six days a week. It's as engrained in us as having a cup of coffee in the morning. It's just what we do.

I personally work out every morning between 8:00 and 10:00 a.m. I rarely schedule anything before 10:00 a.m. No appointments, no phone calls, nothing. Of course, there are days when I have commitments before 10:00, but that is the exception, not the rule.

I travel often with my friend, coaching at her workshops. The workshops run for three days and require long hours working with clients, often until midnight. My friend and I get up every morning of the workshop and go to the hotel gym for a 45-minute workout. I always know she'll be there and she knows I'll be there. In fact, knowing she is going to be there has on occasion prompted me to get my butt up and get to the gym. More so than not, I'll be honest that I'd rather stay in bed for another hour, but here's what I know. Sometime during that afternoon we'll say to each other, "I'm so glad I worked out this morning, I feel so much better now and have much more energy." Never, ever have either of us said, "I wish I'd stayed in bed." Exercise = energy.

Often we use lack of time as an excuse to not eat right. Let's face it; eating healthy fresh food is not as easy as ordering a pizza or opening a bag of chips. Preparing fresh and healthy food takes time, but there are many ways to prepare the right foods to fuel our bodies without making a production out of it. In Chapter 3, "Healthy Eating Habits on a Time Budget," we'll explore ways to plan healthy snacks and meals so you will always have the right kinds of food on hand without a daunting time commitment.

We use the lack-of-time excuse to skip our workouts or exercise. I see this one *a lot*. Once again it goes back to the lack of priority. When we put ourselves and our health and fitness first, not only do we fuel our success, but that success also bleeds over to our business, our family, our friends and all areas of our lives. Getting healthy is the greatest gift we can give to ourselves and all those whose lives we touch. I love the Nike slogan "Just Do It." I've repeated those words over and over in my head

> When we put ourselves and our health and fitness first, not only do we fuel our success, but that success also bleeds over to our business, our family, our friends and all areas of our lives.

when I'm resistant to doing the things I know in my heart I should or must do.

"It's too hard." Damn right it is. Sorry to be so blunt, but let's be frank: what in life really worth having is easy? I don't know of many things. Relationships are hard, running a business is hard, raising kids is hard, but what would our lives be like without these wonderful things? Anything worth having takes work; that's just the way it is. So get off your butt and get to work. Stop the excuses and *Just Do It!*

Regarding diets and weight loss plans, I've heard plenty of excuses as well. The most common complaint (another word for excuse) is that the rate of weight loss is slow. I've experienced that one myself, and boy can it be maddening. You work hard, you follow the program yet the weight just won't come off. Plateaus are part of the process. The trick is to identify a plateau when it rears its ugly head and change things up enough to get off it. In Chapter 6, "Barriers to Success," we'll explore setbacks, plateaus and ways to keep moving forward.

Under normal circumstances, weight loss should be slow, one to two pounds a week is considered safe. Rapid weight loss programs may be satisfying at first, but seldom does the weight stay off. Those kinds of programs can be dangerous and should be avoided.

Many diet and weight loss plans are very restrictive and leave you feeling hungry and deprived. They often work for a short period, but sooner or later you get frustrated or just tired of it. Not only do you go off

> What in life really worth having is easy?

the plan, but you gorge yourself on all the foods you've been missing. Many diets allow you to eat all you want of a small variety of foods. That too gets boring fast and is very hard to adhere to for any length of time.

There are a number of programs out there that work because they prepare your food for you, leaving out any guesswork on what you're consuming. These programs work; I have a dear friend who lost forty pounds on one of them. The problem is that they don't teach you how to eat. Once they quit the program, most people go back to their old eating habits because they haven't replaced their old bad habits with healthy new ones. These programs are expensive and I personally try to avoid eating prepared foods that contain preservatives, chemicals and who knows what else.

These are just some of the excuses I find the most prevalent. We'll explore more excuses and how to overcome them in Chapter 5, "Avoidance and Excuses."

Now that we've talked about all the reasons that you "can't," let's talk about what happens when you commit that you WILL!

Overcoming Obstacles

Whatever the diet, program, or solution you've chosen, you begin with great enthusiasm and focus. For the first couple of days you are solid, maybe for even a whole week. You're sticking to the program and feeling good. Then you hit the first roadblock. Here's what it might look like:

- You hit the gym or begin exercise for the first time in a long time and you over-exert yourself. The next day you're sore and the day after that you experience even more intense soreness, so you quit exercising.
- You make it through the first couple of days but then you slip up. Instead of acknowledging the minor setback, you get frustrated, or mad at yourself and the minor setback becomes a major setback and you quit.

- You're going along fine the first few days or even weeks, but eventually you get bored eating the same foods over and over. You feel deprived of your favorite foods—your comfort foods—so you quit.

- You've been successful until you're faced with one of your challenges. Maybe it's Friday night happy hour, or dinner with your significant other at your favorite restaurant. Maybe it's your friends or colleagues who wish to sabotage your weight loss and in a weak moment you let them.

- You have a family that is not trying to lose weight. You prepare separate meals for them, essentially creating two meals, one for you and one for the family. Now that's really hard, and after a while you quit.

- You've stuck with the program but are not seeing results. Why stick with a program that leaves you feeling deprived and doesn't seem to be working? All this hard work, no results. Quitting time!

- Here's my favorite one. You're an entrepreneur or busy business professional that finds it hard to find the time to eat right or exercise. You start out strong but then the needs of the business or travel start pulling at you. You tell yourself that the business has to come first if it's going to be successful. You put yourself on the back burner until such time as you have more time. Oh, I love this one because that was me for a long time. I convinced myself that my thinking was rational. News flash, your business will never be successful enough and you'll never have enough time unless you change your thought process and behaviors NOW!

> Your business will never be successful enough and you'll never have enough time unless you change your thought process and behaviors NOW!

Keys to Successful Weight Loss

Successful weight loss begins with a commitment to start. The work is hard; sometimes it's not that much fun. You feel deprived because sometimes you have to do things you don't want to do, or skip things you do want to do. In the end though, it's all worth it. Like they say, *"Nothing tastes as good as weight loss feels."*

Once you've made the commitment, the key to successful weight loss is to identify the roadblocks, acknowledge them and have the tools to overcome them. Where do you find the support and tools you need? I believe the answer to that very question is the single most important factor in determining success in weight loss. Let me say that again: I believe the support and tools you receive on your weight loss journey are by far the most significant elements in determining your success.

The support and tools you receive on your weight loss journey are by far the most significant elements in determining your success.

So what does support look like? What tools are available to you to help you to create your success? Support and tools come in a number of different categories.

- **Online tools**. Here are a few examples:
  Weight Watchers: http://www.weightwatchers.com
  Lose It!: http://www.loseit.com
  Livestrong: http://www.livestrong.com
- **Publications.** You'll find countless books available online, in your local bookstore or local library. Topics include:
  o   Nutrition
  o   Wellness
  o   Fitness
  o   Healthy Eating

- º Exercise
- º Fitness Training
- º Weight Loss
- **Support groups.** You'll find many support groups and forums available online. Google the topic you're interested in followed by "forum," for example "weight loss forum." Various in-person support groups are also available; Weight Watchers is the most widespread.
- **Accountability / Coaching.** Accountability is key to success. At the very least, join a support group to help you stay on track and provide accountability—even if the group is just you and a friend. Hire a coach to support you and hold you accountable for the things you say you want. We'll talk more about commitment and accountability in Chapter 9 "Accountability and Commitment."

Along the journey of weight loss and fitness, we encounter habits and beliefs that we hold inside that effect our level of success. In the next chapter, we'll explore the ways in which others attempt to sabotage us, and how we sabotage ourselves.

CHAPTER 1 EXERCISES

What excuses do you use?

_____

_____

_____

_____

What obstacles do you face?

_____

_____

_____

_____

How will you overcome them?

_____

_____

_____

_____

Is it time for you to commit? Yes ____   No ____
Why?

_____

_____

_____

If Yes, congratulations! What actions will you take today to reflect that commitment?

_____

_____

_____

_____

If No, what needs to happen for you to commit?

_____

_____

_____

_____

What does commitment look like for you?

_____

_____

_____

_____

Who will hold you accountable?

_____

_____

_____

_____

What does support look like for you?

_____

_____

_____

_____

You can find these and all the exercise templates on our website at http://www.slimpreneur.com/resources

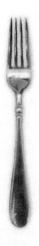

CHAPTER 2:

Self-Sabotage and Other Challenges

Remember, no one can make you feel inferior without your consent.
—**Eleanor Roosevelt**

Begin with Your "Why"

When starting with a new coaching client, we first focus on discovering the client's "Why." It is the first step in determining goals and actions that will lead to success.

Your "Why" is specific to you and everyone's is different. Your "Why" is the single most important underlying reason for your actions.

For many their "Why" is related to their family or loved ones. Much of what they do is a direct result of what they want for themselves and their families. More time together, the freedom

 Your "Why" is the single most important underlying reason for your actions.

to travel, vacation, a better house or home, money to send their children to college, a business they can share with their children, a better life for themselves, their spouse and their children.

A person's "Why" is a powerful motivational force that can help propel them to greatness. People who haven't identified their underlying personal "Why" often flounder, get sidetracked, lose focus and don't reach their goals.

Set SMART Goals

After getting in touch with the "Why," we move on to goal setting. Setting goals leads to achieving goals and ultimate success. The first part of goal setting is determining where you are now. If you don't know where you are, how can you figure out where you want to go? Once you've established your starting point, the next step is to set your goals. Your goals should be "SMART" goals: Specific, Measurable, Attainable, Realistic and Timely.

Specific because the more vague your goals, the less chance you have of achieving them. With weight loss, specific is pretty straightforward: how many pounds you've lost in total or how many pounds lost per week, for example. With fitness, perhaps your goal would be to work out for a certain number of times a week, or for a specific number of hours a week or month.

Weight loss goals that are **measurable** usually include a scale. Daily or weekly weigh-ins will ensure your goals are measurable. With fitness, measureable goals could be if you accomplished the specific goal or not. Perhaps you want to run a five kilometer (5K) race, ride your bike fifty miles or compete in a sprint triathlon. You'll know you accomplished the goal by whether you did it or not.

Any goal, whether it is weight loss, fitness or any other general goal, needs to be **attainable**. Your goals should stretch you, but not be so big a stretch that you can't achieve them, leading to frustration. Frustration leads to quitting and we don't want that. With weight loss the goal could be to lose a certain amount of weight or get into a certain dress or pant size. With fitness, an attainable goal could be to complete a 5K run or work out thirty minutes on the treadmill.

Realistic goals are different from attainable ones in that they are goals you can achieve by your own effort. For example, if you are in your fifty's and want a body of an eighteen-year old, that goal is most likely an unrealistic one. If you've never been a runner, chances are you won't set a world record in your first 10K race. Set goals that, with commitment, focus and some hard work you will achieve. The satisfaction of reaching your goals will encourage you to set bigger goals the next time.

Timely goals are anchored to a time frame. A specific time frame gives you a sense of urgency to complete the task by a specific date. For example, if you've set a goal to lose ten pounds, by when do you want to lose it? "Someday" won't cut it. When you choose a specific date like June 1, you set your wheels in motion and establish a way to gauge your progress. If you set a date to climb a nearby hill or mountain, you know you have to train to be able to achieve that goal on that date. Making your goals "SMART" energetically sets you up for success. You begin firing on all cylinders to make your dreams come true.

> Making your goals "SMART" energetically sets you up for success. You begin firing on all cylinders to make your dreams come true.

Recognize Your Gap

The distance between where you are now and your "SMART" goals is what I refer to as "the Gap." The Gap may be small and it may be gigantic. The size of the Gap, and more importantly the pain caused by the Gap is a source of motivation that can determine your level of success. It is important to identify the Gap and tap into it as a source of inspiration.

You may want to try this exercise. Get out a piece of blank paper. On the left third of the page, describe where you are now. If it's physical changes you want, take a "before" picture or take your measurements. If it's fitness you're after, feel free to use the Fitness Test in the Resources section to assess your current level of fitness. On the right side of the paper write down where you want to be using your "SMART" goals. The white space in the middle of the page is the Gap. You'll find the exercise template at the end of the chapter.

Visualize and then describe on the top middle section of the page what it will be like when you achieve your goals. Be specific: how will your life be different? What things will you be able to do that you couldn't before? What things can you leave behind that haven't been good for you? At the bottom of the middle white space write down what concrete actions you need to do to achieve your goals. Be specific here as well; for example, "I will use my food journal to keep track of my calories," "I commit to going to the gym four days a week," and "I will make good food choices when I'm travelling." Write down the key things that you know you need to do.

Visualize your success; it will help you anchor yourself and get you back on track.

Post your "Gap analysis" somewhere you can see it daily. When hiccups and setbacks occur, and they will, refer back to it. Visualize your success; it will help you anchor yourself and get you back on track.

External Sources of Sabotage

It's an interesting phenomenon, but have you ever noticed that when you get committed to do something that really stretches you, that you really want, people around you try to rain on your parade? Or worse yet, try to sabotage you? It's bad enough how we sabotage ourselves (a topic I'll get to in a minute), but to have our friends, co-workers, family and—Yikes!— spouses or significant others put us down or try to derail our efforts is an outrage. And they can be so stealthy about it. Their subtle comments, such as encouraging us to eat or to skip the gym, simply provoke me. They are supposed to be our support system and often we trust them to stand behind us, only to have them thwart our progress.

I've experienced this in my own life. I once dated a guy who constantly told me that I didn't need to lose weight, that he loved me just the way I am. He would encourage me to eat, which I found blatantly annoying. He would offer to take me out to dinner, knowing full well that I preferred to make my own meals so that I knew exactly what was in them. I work out a lot and did so in those days as well. He would tell me I was overtraining, and that I would injure myself. Once when I pulled a muscle in my leg, and did indeed take a week off, he used that for weeks afterwards saying that I needed more time off, that the injury would come back.

What was his problem? It's my decision whether I need to drop a couple of pounds. It was not like I was at an unhealthy low weight. You'd think he would be encouraging me to get fit. What is it with people who can't seem to give their unconditional support

I believe people are inherently good, but have a little bit of a dark side. People who try to sabotage you do so as a result of their own issues. Much as they say they support you, deep down they don't want you to succeed, because your success is seen as a reflection of their *own* lack of success. Often people just don't want you to change because that change highlights the *lack* of change in their lives. People can be so self-centered at times. So when someone tries to sidetrack your hopes and dreams by steering you off course, recognize it for what it is: their own lack of self worth. Maybe you feel a little sorry for them and move on. Take the high road and know that you're making sound decisions that will get you where you want to go.

People who try to sabotage you do so as a result of their own issues.

Sometimes you have to go as far as to eliminate these negative factors from your life. When I quit my W2 job and embarked on a new career as an entrepreneur, I found a lot of "friends" of mine started to act differently. They told me "You can't" a lot. "You can't just start a career in real estate and become an international land developer." Well, yes you can if you surround yourself with a team who knows what you don't. Many of those folks are no longer in my inner circle. Nowadays I am surrounded by friends and colleagues who get it, who are like-minded, positive and most of all, supportive. I encourage you to do the same. Stop letting in negative influences; they will suck your energy dry. Instead, invite only positive people into your sphere—people who want the same things you want, think the same positive way you do and are there to root for your success.

In my coaching, I often believe in my client's success more than they do. That is part of my role as the coach: to create the space for my clients to grow, to know absolutely they will succeed often before they do. After many years of coaching, I have found that we as humans often undervalue our worth. Some even have friends, family and colleagues that are all too happy to reinforce those thoughts. Our job is to recognize, then dismiss any and all negativity that effects our efforts to achieve what we desire.

Now that we've learned to recognize how the negative thoughts of others affect us, and learned to ignore them, what happens when the negative thoughts come from our own brains?

Self-Sabotage

For many years the focus of my coaching business was in the area of making money and I spent a lot of time with a woman who is known as "The Millionaire Maker." In fact she is one of my best friends. At all of her seminars she begins by challenging the audience to a quiz about their relationship with money. Everyone in the audience is standing and the first statement of the quiz is "If you've had any negative thoughts about money in the last twenty-four hours please sit down." At that point typically about half the audience sits down. I would be surprised if the percentage wasn't much higher if the statement was "If you've had any negative thoughts about yourself in the last twenty-four hours, please sit down."

Negative internal thoughts are very common and can really wreak havoc with your self-esteem. Much of our self perception and negative self talk comes from childhood where at some point we were made to feel we weren't good enough, pretty enough, strong enough, or some other form of not enough. Bad habits die hard. As Julia Roberts says in the movie *Pretty Woman*, "Sometimes it's just easier to believe the bad stuff."

Our internal dialog often arises out of fear, fear of failure, but as I have discovered with my clients, a surprisingly large amount of people actually fear success more. I believe that to be true of weight loss and fitness as well. Weight loss, fitness, better and healthier habits equal change and we as human beings have a basic fear of change. What if the people we love and trust don't like us after we've changed? How will changes that we make in ourselves affect how those around us treat us? This fear keeps us stuck, or we use this fear as a reason not to do the hard work.

The first step to overcoming the fear is to recognize it. Identify it when it comes up, acknowledge it and cast it aside. Look your fear straight in the face and spit in its eye. That's the key to overcoming it.

Look your fear straight in the face and spit in its eye. That's the key to overcoming it.

One of my clients said to me the other day, "No matter how much I've weighed at any time in my life, I've never been happy with my weight." What a sad commentary, to live your life never having been happy with the way you look or the way you feel about your body. I've known this client for a very long time and although she has gained a few pounds in recent years, even when she was very thin, healthy and athletic, she was not happy with her body.

The key to real happiness is accepting who we are both on the inside and outside and being comfortable with our bodies when we are at a healthy weight. Managing expectations are a big part of accepting who we are. Accept yourself just as you are. Change what you need to, but in the end, love yourself.

CHAPTER 2 EXERCISES ✎

Gap Analysis

Where I Am Now	The Gap	Where I Want To Be
	What Will I Be Like When I Achieve My Goals	
	Actions	

What is your Why?

_____

_____

_____

_____

List your SMART Goals
Specific

_____

_____

_____

_____

Measurable

_____

_____

_____

_____

Attainable

_____

_____

_____

_____

Realistic

_____

_____

_____

_____

_____

Timely

_____

_____

_____

_____

List the ways others try to sabotage you.

_____

_____

_____

_____

List your negative self-talk. What negative thoughts do you have?

_____

_____

_____

_____

You can find these and all the exercise templates on our website at http:// www.slimpreneur.com/resources

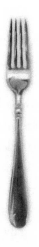

CHAPTER 3:

Healthy Eating Habits on a Time Budget

Diets, like clothes should be tailored to you.
Joan Rivers

Willpower and Restraint

I believe most people think that losing weight means you have to go on a diet. Everybody hates dieting. I know I do. Most people would equate going on a diet with restricting what you eat, eating stuff you don't like, being hungry, depriving yourself and a host of other horrible things. It's true, for most people weight loss will only occur if they change their eating habits. Most likely it's poor eating habits that got them into trouble in the first place. But weight loss doesn't mean you have to go on a diet with all the negative implications of that word. Weight loss and increased fitness can and will occur when you make small changes to your everyday routine.

Recommended Weight Loss and Fitness Tips

Here are some of the tips I'd recommend when you embark on your weight loss and fitness journey. Some may resonate with you; others may not apply to your situation. Take what works for you and leave the rest.

Weight loss and increased fitness can and will occur when you make small changes to your everyday routine.

Clean house. The first thing I'd recommend is that you do a thorough cleaning out of all the junk food you have in your pantry, refrigerator and cupboards. This includes chips, cookies, candy, crackers, ice cream, processed foods and any unhealthy foods that you can't seem to resist. Purge instant meals in a box or a can such as pasta dishes, flavored rice, soups loaded with sodium, and any foods containing trans fats.

A healthy pantry should include cooking staples that allow you to quickly prepare healthy meals. These include olive and canola oil, vinegars for homemade salad dressings and sauces, canned tomatoes, tomato sauce, tomato paste, and canned beans to make sauces, stews and healthy meals rich in fiber. Nuts make a great snack—have them on hand. Brown rice and quinoa are good staples to always keep in your pantry. Fiber-rich cereals, stock for soups and stews, and whole-wheat pastas are also good for easy, quick meals.

Eat five times a day. I believe in eating five times a day as opposed to three main meals. I recommend three smaller main meals and two snacks. The purpose behind eating smaller meals more frequently is to maintain a steady supply of glucose to the blood stream therefore preventing the large fluctuations in blood sugar normally associated with the traditional three large meals a day. Eating every couple of hours keeps your sugar levels steady, which keeps energy levels constant without spikes or dips.

Admittedly there are a couple of downsides to the "Eat five times a day" strategy. Sitting down to five meals a day as opposed to three may lead to overeating. Be careful that you are not eating more in the five meals than you would normally consume in three meals.

The goal in eating smaller meals more frequently is to maintain blood sugar and prevent hunger. Going several hours without eating often leads to eating more when you finally do sit down to a meal. Avoid that scenario. Eating five small meals takes time, and for the busy business professional, time is precious. Planning is the key to success here. Keep plenty of healthy snacks on hand and available, particularly when you travel. Check out the list of quick and easy foods for travel in the Resources section in the back of the book. I've included a list of the foods I take on the road with me to make sure I stay on my healthy eating plan.

Follow the 30-30-40 rule. Adhere to a good, healthy eating plan that includes a recommended proportion of 30 percent protein, 30 percent healthy fat and 40 percent complex carbohydrates. For example if your daily calorie intake is 2000 calories, aim for 500 calories for breakfast, lunch and dinner. Then add two snacks between those meals that amount to approximately 250 calories each. Make sure each meal or snack contains a good balance of protein, fat and carbohydrates. When you follow this strategy you'll find you are seldom hungry and feel energized throughout the day. Be sure to include protein in every meal or snack. Protein is sometime difficult to include so here are some suggestions for ways to add healthy sources of protein.

- Protein Powder
- Turkey or Beef Jerky
- Non-Fat Cottage Cheese
- Eggs or Egg Whites
- Soy Protein
- Hard Cheeses

- Beans
- Edamame
- Yogurt
- Chicken or Turkey Breast
- Peanut Butter

Keep healthy snacks on hand. Nothing will derail your weight loss efforts faster than being hungry and not having access to healthy snacks. Now that you've cleaned out your pantry, it's time to replace those foods with healthy, fresh foods and snacks. Some of my favorites include nuts, yogurt with fruit, protein shakes, cottage cheese, fresh fruits and vegetables, and hard-boiled eggs. I carry them with me when I travel. In fact, I have a whole travel food strategy that I'll share with you later in the chapter.

Always having good snacks on hand can require some planning and preparation. I like to cook, but don't always have the time. When I do cook, usually on the weekends, whatever I make always includes lots of vegetables. I like my dishes to contain lots of bright colors that come from healthy vegetables. During meal preparation I cut up extra vegetables that I can snack on during the week. I store them in small Tupperware containers that I can take with me on the go. I hard-boil eggs while I'm preparing dinner so I don't have to make a special effort. With minimal effort, I always have good-for-me snacks available.

Eat your vegetables first. This is a trick I learned during my time with Weight Watchers. First of all, I always make sure that my meals consist of plenty of colorful, healthy and fresh vegetables. Steamed vegetables by the way, not ones laden with butter, oil or sauces. When I sit down to eat I always eat all my vegetables first. I still do this today, a habit my friends find a little strange, but heck, it

Eating your veggies first helps fill you up with healthy low-calorie food that's good for you and ensures you get your daily allotment of fresh vegetables.

works. These days I do it without even recognizing that I'm doing it, it's such an engrained habit. Eating your veggies first helps fill you up with healthy low-calorie food that's good for you and ensures you get your daily allotment of fresh vegetables.

Drink plenty of water. When my friends and I were in Weight Watchers, they drilled into our heads the need to drink lots of water. Certain weeks where we didn't lose what we thought we should, it often was because we hadn't had enough water.

To this day, I drink tons of water. Not juice, not coffee or diet soda, but plain old water. I aim for 64 ounces of water a day and often drink more than that. I don't include in my 64 ounces the water I drink while working out, the tea I drink in the morning or any other fluids I might consume throughout the day. I only count plain water that I drink out of a 32-ounce water bottle that I always carry with me.

There are tons of benefits to drinking water. The body is made up of more than 50 percent water. The water in your body transports nutrients and oxygen to your cells. Water helps with metabolism, regulates body temperature and detoxifies.

If you don't have enough water in your body, it will not function well. Think of your body as your employee. If you don't pay your employee, i.e. give it good food and plenty of water, it will stop working for you. If you are asking a lot of your body, for example when you exercise, how do expect your body/employee to work harder if you don't pay it more? Some of the health benefits of drinking plenty of water include:

- *Weight Loss.* Drinking water helps you lose weight because it flushes your body of the by-products produced by the breakdown of fat and reduces hunger so you'll eat less.
- *Fatigue Relief.* Water flushes toxins and waste out of the body. If you don't have enough water to flush out the bad stuff, your body will have to work harder to get rid of it, tiring your body out and leading to fatigue.

- *Headache Relief.* Drinking plenty of water can help to relieve a headache brought on by dehydration.
- *Younger Skin.* Drinking water gives you younger and healthier looking skin.
- *Better Brain Power.* Your brain is 90 percent water so drinking ample amounts of water keeps you thinking clearly, more alert and focused.
- *Better Exercise Performance.* Water helps regulate your body temperature and fuels your muscles which means you'll have more energy for your workouts.
- *Less Cramping or Injuries.* Water keeps your muscles and joints lubricated so you're less prone to injury.
- *Reduce the Risk of Cancer.* Some studies have shown that drinking the recommended amount of water can reduce bladder and colon cancer by diluting the concentration of cancer causing agents in the urine while reducing the time they come in contact with the lining of the bladder.

Write it down! Successful weight loss comes with a combination of eating a certain amount of calories per day and exercise. It really is as simple as that. Simple, but not easy.

Counting calories is the best way I know of to ensure you stick to your weight loss plan. Many of my clients complain about writing everything down. "It takes too long, it's a pain in the butt," they say. I agree with all that; nevertheless, it remains the best tool for consistent, successful weight loss.

Back in my days of Weight Watchers, I kept a food journal. I bought all the books that told me how many calories, fat, protein and fiber were in each food. I also purchased books that told me the point value of many foods. (For more information about Weight Watchers Points Plan, visit their website at http://www.weightwatchers.com)

Today it is much easier to track the foods that you eat. There are online programs and smart phone apps with extensive food databases that make it fast and simple to keep track. I encourage anyone looking to lose weight to start by keeping track of the calories they consume. After some time you get to know the calories in most of the food that you eat and you can keep track without writing everything

Be careful that you don't add additional calories because you're not keeping a food journal. Be honest with yourself.

down. Just be careful that you don't add additional calories because you're not keeping a food journal. Be honest with yourself.

Get plenty of sleep. We all know that getting eight hours of sleep is good for us, but did you know that recent studies have shown that sleep can affect our appetite? Studies report that inadequate sleep reduces the levels of the hormone leptin that signals satisfaction to the brain. Conversely, sleep deprivation increases levels of the hormone ghrelin, which stimulates the sense of hunger to the brain. Try to keep a consistent sleep schedule that includes seven to nine hours of sleep per night. I find that exercise enhances my ability to sleep and the quality of my rest. Routine exercise enhances my ability to get a good night's sleep.

Have an "On the Go" travel strategy. I mentioned I have a whole strategy that I use when I travel. I tailor my strategy for travel by car or travel by plane and by length of stay.

When I travel by car for a day trip and I know will not have access to food or the food choices won't work with my plan, I pack a small, insulated lunch bag with meals and snacks. I'll make a sandwich, or half sandwich with whole grain bread and turkey meat and light or soy cheese slices. Sometimes I make a sandwich without the bread using lettuce leaves. I pack a small container with mustard or light mayonnaise. I love cut-up carrots with peanut butter; I know it sounds strange, but try it! I'll pack a banana, an apple, grapes or other fresh fruit for snacks. I like to have turkey jerky or light string cheese with me to make sure I get enough protein.

I always carry a PowerBar with me for emergencies. If I find myself at a meeting or event where the food provided is not the healthy food I'd prefer to eat, instead of caving in and eating what's there, I eat my PowerBar with lots of water. It's a good alternative that will satisfy you in a pinch. I prefer PowerBars, but any energy bar you like that contains around 30 percent protein, 40 percent carbohydrate and 30 percent fat in 250 calories or less is good.

For longer trips in the car I bring a cooler and fill it with healthy food I can rely on to keep me on track. In addition to the meals and snacks I mentioned above, I'll add hard-boiled eggs, cottage cheese and yogurt. If I know I'll have access to a microwave I'll even bring individual sized frozen meals left over from dishes I've prepared prior to my trip.

I'm always thinking of ways to prepare and save healthy food for my busy on-the-go lifestyle. It's easy if you think ahead and plan. I have some favorite dishes that I discovered along the way that I still make today.

One of the favorites is my "100-Calorie Chili." It packs a ton of satisfying goodness in a small amount of calories. It's tasty and filling, low in fat, high in complex carbohydrates, protein and fiber. I make a big batch of the chili that we'll have on a cold winter evening, then I'll freeze the rest in single-serving containers. They're great for taking on trips where you can bring along a cooler.

The key is to identify a couple of your favorite recipes, then when you make them, prepare extra and freeze in single-serving amounts. You'll never be without a healthy alternative when you're on the road. You can find this recipe and many other healthy and delicious recipes in the Resources section in the back of the book.

I'm always thinking of ways to prepare and save healthy food for my busy on-the-go lifestyle. It's easy if you think ahead and plan.

The most challenging of travel scenarios is air travel. Even then I have a few tricks up my sleeve. I always carry something to eat on the plane, regardless of my destination. The food choices in airports are notoriously bad and I refuse to blow a week's worth of progress on airport food that doesn't taste very good anyway.

I carry on to the plane a meal and enough snacks to get me through the flight so that I don't arrive hungry and ready to eat a house. Some of my favorite take-along foods include a healthy sandwich, cheese sticks, nuts, cut-up veggies, 100-calorie fiber bars and fruit for dessert. I pack enough to get me through the flight but no so much that I eat all the way to my destination. Remember the point of bringing your own food is to keep you nourished with healthy food while keeping you from being hungry.

In my luggage, I pack food for my stay. I find that breakfast is the most challenging meal of the day while I'm on the road. I would rather spend my time in the morning in the hotel gym or running outside so I rarely make time for breakfast in the hotel restaurant. Often I travel to events that provide some form of breakfast; rarely is it anything I'm willing to eat. It would appear that donuts, bagels, croissants and muffins are a lot cheaper than eggs, fruit or oatmeal.

Remember the point of bringing your own food is to keep you nourished with healthy food while keeping you from being hungry.

That's why I bring my own and make breakfast in my room. I always carry green tea and start my day with that. Most of the rooms I stay in have a coffee maker so I can heat water and stir up my own instant oatmeal. I prefer the low-sugar brands that I sweeten with dried fruit. Add a sprinkling of nuts and you have a healthy and nutritious breakfast you can whip up in a hurry that will keep you satisfied.

A word on breakfast: I never, ever skip breakfast. It is by far the most important meal of the day and sets the tone for the rest of your day. It jump starts your metabolism and gives you energy for clear thought. Skip

> Skip breakfast and you'll pay for it for the remainder of your day. You'll be sluggish, tired and worst of all, hungry.

breakfast and you'll pay for it for the remainder of your day. You'll be sluggish, tired and worst of all, hungry. By the time lunch comes around you're famished and ready to eat whatever you can get your hands on. Plan ahead and you'll never have to start your day without fuel again.

Lasting Change

The key to success in anything you do is determined by your level of commitment and willingness to change. Weight loss and fitness are no exception. What we're talking about here is lifetime change, not just situational change. While weight loss is not easy, the challenge often comes after the weight is off: how do you keep it off? Lasting change only comes when we teach ourselves new habits that stay with us long after the pounds have melted away.

While I don't endorse any specific weight loss plan, I do believe the ones that teach you how to eat for the rest of your life are by far the most effective. Enrolling in a program that provides ready-made meals right to

> Lasting change only comes when we teach ourselves new habits that stay with us long after the pounds have melted away.

your door—while convenient and less work than counting every calorie—does little to prepare you for the day you stop the program. These types of programs do not teach you how to eat properly, so your chances of gaining the weight back plus some is exceptionally high.

To create permanent change on the outside, there must be a shift of belief on the inside. This is why people who lose weight often gain it all back. They use willpower and determination to starve themselves, which works for a while. They don't change the "program" and self-image that lead them to gain weight in the first place. We'll explore this in more depth in Chapter 8, "Changing the Way You Think Will Change the Way You Look." Next, let's explore the role of exercise in having the life of your dreams.

CHAPTER 3 EXERCISES

List at least five weight loss or fitness tips you will commit to starting today.
You can use the ones listed in the book or create your own.

_____

_____

_____

_____

_____

_____

_____

_____

_____

List your favorite healthy foods and snacks.

_____

_____

_____

_____

If you travel, list your On The Go travel plan foods.

_____

_____

_____

_____

You can find these and all the exercise templates on our website at http://www.slimpreneur.com/resources

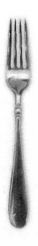

CHAPTER 4:

Fast, Effective Exercise for Weight Loss and Fitness

Don't compromise yourself. You are all you've got.
—Janis Joplin

W e've all heard that the key to weight loss and fitness is diet and exercise. Changing your eating habits is essential for weight loss. Combine that with exercise and you'll reach your goals faster while getting fit.

Start From Where You Are

As with any aspiration in life, before you can move towards it you must first assess where you are. If weight loss is your goal, weighing yourself is a good first step. While it seems an obvious initial step in the process, for some of us, it's not as easy as just stepping on the scale. I know I've suffered from the "stick my head in the sand" syndrome. You may know what I mean: not getting on the scale because you don't want to know what it says.

Getting on the scale and seeing the reality of weight gain can be daunting for some. I know I've avoided the stark truth in the past. Just to share with you the extent I've taken it, I've actually said to myself, "I'll get on the scale after I've lost a few pounds so the reality isn't quite so harsh."

I've learned from experience that the truth is the truth so stop hiding and face the music! If you know you've gained weight, weighing yourself is the first step to taking the pounds off. What are you waiting for?

> If you know you've gained weight, weighing yourself is the first step to taking the pounds off.

If you're concerned about your weight, there are several ways to determine if you are overweight. Here's the most fundamental: unless you're suffering from an eating disorder or have body image issues, if you think you need to lose weight, you most likely do. Regarding eating disorders: we don't touch on that subject in this book. If you suspect you have an eating disorder, please seek professional help immediately.

Another way to understand your ideal weight is to use a chart like the one below to determine if your weight is within the desired range.

Ideal Weight Chart

Height	Minimum For All Adults (17+)	Recommended upper target for ages 17 to 25 years	Recommended upper target for ages 26 to 45 years	Maximum for all Adults over 45 years
4'9"	92	106	111	116
4'10"	96	110	115	120
4'11"	99	114	119	124
5'0"	102	118	123	128
5'1"	106	121	127	132

5'2"	109	125	131	137
5'3"	113	130	135	141
5'4"	117	134	140	146
5'5"	120	138	144	150
5'6"	124	142	148	155
5'7"	128	147	153	160
5'8"	132	151	158	164
5'9"	135	155	162	169
5'10"	139	160	167	174
5'11"	143	165	172	179
6'0"	147	169	177	184
6'1"	152	174	182	189
6'2"	156	179	187	195
6'3"	160	184	192	200
6'4"	164	189	197	205
6'5"	169	194	202	211

Another tool typically used to assess whether you are overweight is the Body Mass Index or BMI. Recommended by the National Institute of Health, BMI uses your weight and height to estimate what percent of your body weight is made up of fat. It provides a measure of your risk for developing the kinds of diseases that are more common when the body stores more fat. The higher your BMI, the higher your risk for heart disease, high blood pressure, type 2 diabetes, breathing problems and certain types of cancers.

BMI Chart

You can use the BMI chart in the Resources section in the back of the book, or log on to http://www.bmi-calculator.net to calculate your BMI. Once you have your BMI, use the chart below to determine your BMI score:

	BMI
Underweight	Below 18.5
Normal	18.5 – 24.9
Overweight	25.0 – 29.9
Obese	30.0 and Above

Now that you know where you are, let's figure out what kind of exercises best fit your lifestyle. Study after study has proven that activity promotes weight loss and fitness. Exercise combined with improved eating habits help the pounds come off faster. More importantly, exercise is essential for keeping the weight off.

Before you begin any exercise program, you'll want to make sure you are prepared. The questionnaire below asks some simple questions that will help ensure you are ready to begin.

Activity Readiness Questionnaire

	Yes	No
Have you ever been told by a doctor that you have a heart condition or problem of any kind?		
Have you ever experienced chest pain during physical activity?		
Have you ever experienced fainting spells or dizziness?		
Are any of your bones or joints bothered by physical exercise?		
Do you have any sore bones or joints?		
Are you taking any medications for high blood pressure or a heart condition?		
Are you aware of any other physical problem you may have that could affect your ability to start exercising?		

If you answered Yes to any of the questions above or have been sedentary for an extended length of time, check with your physician before starting any kind of exercise program.

Create Your Plan

Once you've decided you are ready to begin an exercise program, the next step is to choose an activity you'll enjoy and stick with. If you are a beginner, you will want to start slowly. Many an exercise plan has been derailed by someone starting off too fast and being too sore to exercise for days after the first workout.

Make sure your exercise plan fits into your busy schedule. I've found this can be the biggest impediment to sticking with your program. Determine your exercise plan, put it on your calendar, enlist friends and family to workout with, hire a personal trainer, make a commitment to follow your workout plan, and reward yourself when you do.

Sometimes it even helps to play games with yourself. Last winter I was saving to buy a kayak. I could have easily just put money aside every month until I had the money I needed to buy the kayak. Instead, I made a deal with myself: for every day I ate right and worked out, I'd put $10 in a jar. By June I had a brand new kayak and was in great shape. I even went as far as to put gold stars on my calendar for each day I successfully achieved my goal. You should have seen that calendar—gold stars were everywhere. I don't know why it is, but for me the visual example of all my hard work was empowering.

Types of Exercise

There are three basic types of physical activity: aerobic, resistance training and stretching.

Aerobic or cardiovascular (sometimes referred to as cardio) uses the large muscles of the body to burn calories and improve overall fitness. Examples include walking, running, biking, swimming, and aerobic dance.

Resistance training, sometimes referred to as weight training, uses dumbbells or other forms of weights, resistance bands, weight lifting machines or the weight of your own body. This type of training strengthens, tones, builds muscles, and improves bone density and posture. While often people think weight lifting requires working out in a gym, there are plenty of resistance exercises that you can do at home or while traveling.

Although many people don't consider **stretching** physical activity, it is an integral component of any exercise plan. Stretching includes bending, flexing and elongating the muscles to improve flexibility and range of motion, relieving tight muscles and very importantly, preventing injury. Don't skip the stretching part of your workouts. Yoga, Pilates, martial arts, or basic stretching exercises should become part of your workout routine.

Exercise Intensity Levels

You've planned your workout schedule and perhaps some good-for-you rewards. You've identified the types of activities you want to include in your fitness plan. Now it's time to get to work. But just how hard should you work? What's your intensity level? There are three levels of intensity–light, moderate and high.

- During a light-intensity activity, you should be able to talk, sing, and breathe regularly, and you should not break a sweat.
- During a moderate-intensity activity, you can talk but not sing. You should experience deep breathing and break a sweat after ten minutes of activity.
- During a high-intensity activity, you should be able to talk, but only briefly, and not be able to sing. Your breathing should be rapid and deep, and you should break a sweat three to five minutes into the exercise.

Remember if you are just starting out, start with light intensity and increase it as you become more comfortable with the activity.

Don't forget to warm up and cool down! Before immediately engaging in an activity, take a few moments to warm up, especially in the morning hours just after getting out of bed and in colder weather. Warming up your muscles will help blood flow, allow your muscles to perform at their best and prevent injury. Warm up for at least five minutes before beginning any activity.

After completing your workout, be sure to include time for your body to cool down. Slow down your activity and do as the name implies: let your body temperature, heart rate and blood pressure return to normal. Allow at least five minutes of cool-down after any activity. The more intense the activity, the longer the cool-down may take. Your cool-down is a good time to do some stretching. Your body will love you for it.

The number and duration of your workouts should depend on your fitness level. For beginners, ten to fifteen minutes of moderate activity may be a good start. As you increase your level of fitness you'll increase the length, intensity and frequency of your workouts. Moderately fit to athletic exercisers should work out four to six times a week and include aerobic, resistance training and stretching for optimal results, whether the goal is to lose weight or just get into better shape.

As you increase your level of fitness, you'll increase the length, intensity and frequency of your workouts.

Fitness Test

You may find our Fitness Test helpful in determining your level of fitness and as a way to track your progress. Simply take the test at the beginning of your fitness program and at regular intervals as you progress. I suggest you retest every thirty to sixty days. Recording your progress is one of the best ways to make sure you stay on track. It can also be a great motivator. You can find the Fitness Test in the Resources section in the back of the book, or at our website http://www.slimpreneur.com/resources.

Often just finding the time to work out can be a challenge for the busy entrepreneur or business professional. I find working out can be particularly challenging while I'm traveling. I use many of the same strategies on the road as I do at home. I put my workouts on my calendar. I make a commitment to a certain number of workouts while I'm traveling. I get up early to get my workouts in. And when I really don't want to get up, I tell myself I'll get up and do ten minutes—that's it, just ten minutes, then I can stop. What I find is, once I'm up and exercising, I do my whole workout, not just a part of it. I have a friend Sam that I see in the gym almost every day. He has great dedication to fitness and working out. I asked him his strategy for getting to the gym every day. He said, "Not every day has to be your best day." I love that.

When I really don't want to get up, I tell myself I'll get up and do ten minutes—that's it, just ten minutes, and then I can stop. What I find is, once I'm up and exercising, I do my whole workout, not just a part of it.

If you find yourself on the road without a workout facility, don't use that as an excuse to skip a workout. I've developed a simple workout program that is specifically designed for times when no gym is available. I designed this workout so that it could be done in a hotel room or any limited space. All you'll need is a set of exercise or resistance bands. They're inexpensive and you can find them online or in any sporting goods store, Target or Walmart. You can find the Travel Strength Training Workout in the Resources section in the back of the book or on our website http://www.slimpreneur.com/resources.

I also find that I feel so much better for the rest of the day when I work out. Even when I'm really tired, I find that a workout in the morning energizes me for the whole day. Not once have I ever said to myself, I wish I hadn't gotten up this morning and worked out.

Well let's face it, getting up and working out every day is not always reality. There are days we turn off the alarm and go back to bed. We promise ourselves we'll work out later in the day and it just doesn't happen. So what, we've all done it. Don't beat yourself up for it. Acknowledge it and get right back to it the next day. Too many people use falling off the wagon as an excuse to never to get back up again. Don't let that be you. You owe it to yourself to be the fittest and healthiest you can be.

CHAPTER 4 EXERCISES

List your favorite exercises.

_____

_____

_____

_____

_____

_____

_____

_____

Commit to a fitness/workout plan. When will you start? Write it down.

_____

_____

_____

_____

_____

Record your workout schedule, number of days a week, exercises, duration, and so on.

_____

_____

_____

_____

_____

_____

_____

_____

_____

_____

Congratulate yourself for a job well done!

You can find these and all the exercise templates on our website at http://www.slimpreneur.com/resources

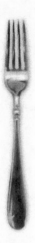

CHAPTER 5:

Avoidance and Excuses

Mistakes are part of the dues one pays for a full life.
—Sophia Loren

Avoidance and Body Checking

Janet Latner of the Department of Psychology at the University of Hawaii conducted a study called *Body Checking and Avoidance Among Behavioral Weight-Loss Participants*. The study found a correlation between obesity and what she refers to as body checking and avoidance. The study goes on to connect low self-esteem with participants in the study who were significantly overweight. Duh! I never really knew it had a scientific name but I am familiar with body checking and avoidance.

Have you ever found yourself wearing oversized clothes so no one can see your body? Have you ever avoided tight clothes because you didn't like the way your body looked in them? Have you ever pulled your shirt or sweater away from your body so it didn't cling to you? Have you ever moved certain articles of clothing to the back of the closet, "to wear when I lose ten pounds?" Have you ever avoided looking in mirrors, or looking at yourself naked? Have you ever wanted to be intimate, but only in the dark?

If you've ever experienced any of these, you know all about body checking and avoidance. Although I appreciate the hard work and research that went into the report by Ms. Latner, I didn't need an entire study to know that feeling fat, or having a low body image leads to behaviors such as body checking and avoidance.

I'll be honest: I've exhibited some of those behaviors in the past. As I was jotting down ideas for this book, one of the topics I included was to talk about the habit of pulling clothes away from your body when you feel self-conscious about your weight, a habit I have been known to exhibit and have often seen others do as well. Little did I know, until I did a Google search on it, that so many others exhibited the behavior that they did a complete study on it.

I read the entire study and found the results and conclusions to be completely obvious. When you don't feel good about the way you look, you mirror those feelings in the way you act. You avoid, you cover up, and sometimes you fixate on the things you can't stand about yourself. Although the study didn't take it this far, I know that the more you fixate on the things you dislike about yourself, the more of them you'll get.

I have a friend who constantly touches her stomach as she talks about how chubby it is. I keep telling her, "Yes and it will stay that way as long as you tell yourself that you have a fat stomach." The study showed that people who obsessed about

When you don't feel good about the way you look, you mirror those feelings in the way you act.

being fat lost the least amount of weight—perhaps because they gave up, or perhaps because they got exactly what they believed: that they were fat.

Avoidance and body checking are only symptoms of how we feel about ourselves. These thoughts and feelings can spur us on or they can hold us back. It all depends on what we do with them. Let's look at a few illustrative examples (with fictional names).

Judy has a few pounds to lose. She doesn't quite fit into her clothes like she used to, and feels self-conscious wearing most of her outfits. Instead of going out and buying the next size bigger jeans or oversized sweaters to cover up her body, Judy fights back. She assesses what got her to where she is today—what actions and behaviors led to her gaining the additional weight. She puts together a game plan that includes scheduled workouts and healthy meals, and then she gets after it. She doesn't deprive herself or expect immediate results. She goes back to basics and gets the weight off.

Sara is one who has always battled her weight and has slowly put on more and more pounds over the years. Her closet is a mix of different sizes—10, 12, 14, 16—reflecting her slow weight gain over several years. Sara's body checking and avoidance is at an all-time high. She is shocked when she sees a photo of herself. Faced with the reality of who she has become, she decides it's time to make a change. She finds a support team to help her and educate her on what it takes to be healthy and fit. Her weight loss journey has begun and she will be successful.

Finally there's Brenda, who could be either Judy or Sara, but lacks the commitment to change. Brenda feels sorry for herself with a million excuses as to why she can't lose the weight. She is so far in avoidance that she can't see her way out. She gives up because she doesn't think she can change, or she's just afraid to try. She has yet to reach the point where the pain of staying where she is has become greater than moving forward, however scary that may seem.

I've been in situations like that, where the prospect of moving forward is so daunting that you stay stuck where you are. In times like that I ask the following questions. What's it worth to you? Do you really want to stay where you are? Is it worth it to you to continue with the behaviors that are causing you to *fail* in getting what you want? What is worth more to you, eating that chocolate cake or losing that pound and moving forward towards the life you want to have?

What's more important? Ask yourself: Is being afraid and living the status quo more important than getting what you want? Is the fear of failure or committing to some hard work more important than your health and fitness and feeling awesome about yourself?

What's it worth to you? Do you really want to stay where you are? Is it worth it to you to continue with the behaviors that are causing you to *fail* in getting what you want?

What do you want more? During the struggle for weight loss, sometimes it comes down to a test of wills. It comes down to a choice, what do you want more? I've faced this challenge when confronted with social engagements where I know there will be food and wine that I will be tempted to consume. I love wine by the way. At moments like that I have to ask myself, "What do I want more," wine or weight loss?" For me personally I have to prepare myself for the battle before I enter the ring so that I have a clear game plan for choosing a healthier alternative.

One of my favorite sayings is, "no food tastes as good as being slim feels." For me that just about says it all. If I fear that the challenge may get the better of me, I will skip that social outing altogether, knowing there will always be more. I'm clear on what I want.

A Million Excuses—Okay, Twenty-Five

We all make excuses from time to time. It's human nature; it's what we do. The most common reason behind excuses is to get out of doing something we don't want to do, like eating a healthy diet and exercising. Here are some of the basic reasons we make excuses:

- It's just plain easier to make excuses
- We are busy and have limited time

- Our priorities are out of sync
- Why do today what we can put off till tomorrow?
- We are impatient
- We love instant gratification
- There's always something we'd rather do
- We don't know how to begin
- We don't have goals or the ones we have don't serve us
- We don't believe the benefits will outweigh the costs
- We love the role of victim
- We think we are already healthy enough
- Denial is a great state
- We're sporting a negative attitude
- We ignore the pain (of not getting into our favorite jeans)
- We lack commitment
- We don't want to do the work; that is, we're lazy

I hear excuses all the time as they pertain to weight loss and fitness. Here's a list of the most common ones and what you can do to overcome them.

I don't have the time.
- Time management. Look at what you are doing now and how you are spending your time. What things can you eliminate? What things can you hire someone else to do? Most likely those things are things you don't like to do or are not very good at anyway.
- Set your priorities. Take a good look at what's most important in your day. If your health and fitness are not near or at the top of your list, reassess. They should be.
- Look for ways to combine activities; take a brisk walk or run while taking the dog out or exercise while watching TV. Watching TV or reading while exercising decreases the chance you'll challenge

yourself and get a good workout so I don't usually recommend it, but it's better than no exercise at all.

- My favorite, make an exercise appointment with yourself and keep it!
- Plan your day. Employ good time management skills and plan time to workout.

Twenty minutes of exercise is better than none at all.

- Get up thirty minutes earlier.
- Remember twenty minutes of exercise is better than none at all.
- Park far away from your destination and walk.
- Take the stairs.
- Plan, plan, and plan. Whether you're scheduling time to work out or organizing healthy meals for the week, planning is the key.

I have too many other obligations.

- Change your priorities and let those around you know what your priorities are so that they can support you.
- Your weight loss and fitness goals are very important to you and your overall health—don't forget that.
- Keep your goals close at hand to remind you of what is important to you.
- Simplify. Sometimes we try to do too much. Simplify your life if you can.

I can't do it alone.

- You don't have to. Hire a personal trainer. If you're on a budget, hire a personal trainer for one or two sessions to show you some basic exercises and ensure you have good form, then continue on your own.
- Join a gym. If they have organized classes there, take some classes. Meet new people who share your desire to get fit.

- Work out with a friend. Walk with a co-worker at lunchtime or after work. Go to the gym together. If you both are trying to lose weight, start your own support group, even if it's just the two of you. Share challenges and successes.
- Join a weight loss organization like Weight Watchers and attend weekly meetings.
- Educate yourself by reading articles on weight loss and fitness.
- Join an online forum. Many weight loss and fitness websites have free forums where you can sign up and participate in live chats, exchange recipes, log workouts and interact with like-minded people.

I don't get enough support at home.

- For many, having support is the key to achieving their weight loss and fitness goals. If you aren't getting the support you need at home, seek it elsewhere. There are lots of organizations there to support you.

- You'll find those around you will become more supportive when they know you are serious and see the work you are putting into getting what you want.

> You'll find those around you will become more supportive when they know you are serious and see the work you are putting into getting what you want.

- Get started anyway and the support will come. When they see your commitment and determination, you'll find your family is anxious to support you.
- If you still aren't getting the support you need at home, do it anyway. Don't let the lack of support keep you from success in getting what you want.

I'm hurt or injured.

- We all suffer injuries at one time or another and we all experience pain. The key is to find a way to continue to get the exercise you need, working around your injury.
- Find an exercise you can do. If you can't run, walk briskly. If you can't walk, get into the pool and swim. Find something that you can do to move your body and work up a sweat.
- Keep moving. Any activity burns calories, so stay in movement.
- Visit a sports medicine doctor and ask him or her to prescribe exercises that you can do without aggravating your injury.
- Try stretching or yoga, or a resistance band workout. Any physical activity that increases your heart rate will consume energy and help you burn calories.
- Just because you're injured doesn't mean you can ignore your diet. In fact, just the opposite is true. When you're injured, you may be working out less and burning fewer calories. Make sure you take that into consideration and compensate by eating right.

I don't feel good.

- Nothing will make you feel better than a good workout and healthy eating. It's true that physical exercise releases endorphins that improve your mood. That combined with becoming more physically fit will do wonders to improve how you feel.

> Physical exercise releases endorphins that improve your mood. That combined with becoming more physically fit will do wonders to improve how you feel.

- Eating right will give you all the nutrients you need to fuel your body and clear your mind.

- If you don't feel like working out, tell yourself you just need to start and only do five minutes. Chances are, once you are geared up and begin an exercise routine, you won't quit after five minutes. The hardest part is to begin.

I'm too out of shape.

- Okay, and your point is what? I'm too out of shape to do anything to get into shape? One of the worst excuses on the planet.
- Start slow with simple exercises at low intensity.
- Get out and walk. Even if it is a walk to the mailbox and back, just get out there and start. Increase your distance a little each day.

I'm too stressed out.

- Another of my favorite excuses. Guess what? Exercise reduces stress! Eating right reduces the stresses on your body.
- Just start. Some of the stress you feel may come from the fact that you know you should be doing good things for your health and you're not. Start today.

I'm too busy taking care of my spouse and kids.

- And if you're too sick or unhealthy to take care of them who will?
- Incorporate them into your exercise routine. If you have very small children, walk or run with their stroller. Take your kids to the park and play with them. Walk, run, hike or swim with your kids.
- Include healthy meals for you and for all of your family.
- Get creative with new healthy and fun recipes.

I get enough exercise at work.

- Although you may be active at work, the exercise you get may not the right kind or fit in with your fitness plans. Maintain a well-balanced fitness routine to ensure you're getting a good balance of cardio and strength training.

I'm too tired.

- Believe it or not, exercise perks you up and makes you feel less tired. Just get out there and move.
- Exercise increases the quality and quantity of your sleep.
- Exercise may make you feel tired, but after a couple of weeks your body will adjust and you will have more energy than before you began an exercise routine.

Hormones are giving me problems.

- Exercise and good nutrition can combat the effects of hormones.
- Exercise and healthy eating practices can help to stabilize your hormone levels.

I don't want to go outside, it's too hot or cold or it's raining.

- If the weather is preventing you from exercising outdoors, go to a gym, an indoor pool or track, or exercise at home.
- If you live where the weather is blistering hot, exercise in the morning or the evening before or after the heat of the day. Exercise in an air-conditioned space.
- If it's cold outside, dress in layers that will keep you warm, and that can be shed as your body warms up.

I'm bored with exercising.

- Get over it. Exercise is not supposed to entertain you; it's supposed to get or keep you fit, healthy and happy.
- Find an activity that you like to do. There has to be something that gets you to move that you can enjoy.
- Exercise with a friend.
- Take an exercise class. The energy of others will propel you along.
- Try something new, like a dance class, rollerblading or snowshoeing.
- Listen to your favorite music while exercising. I like to put together play lists that include slower songs for the warm up

and cool down and a combination of fast and ultra fast songs for interval training.

- Use your MP3 player on shuffle. I like to let my iPod determine the speed of my walk, run, bike, elliptical or workout. I tailor the speed of my movements to the speed of the song that comes on.
- Change up your routine. Do different exercises each day. One day, you might run or walk. Another day you might ride your bike or rollerblade. The key is to vary your routines. This will not only keep you from getting bored, it will keep your body guessing—which leads to better results.
- The fitter and stronger you become, the more you will enjoy and appreciate exercise.

I'm too overweight to exercise.

- Speak to a physician before starting any form of exercise.
- Start out slowly. If walking around the block is all you can do to start, then begin there. Go easy at first and increase the length of time or intensity gradually as your body adapts.
- Focus on eating a healthy and nutritious diet. As you start to lose weight, slowly add exercise.

I can't afford a gym or a personal trainer.

- Personal trainers are great if you can afford them, but if you can't, don't fret. There are other ways to learn how to exercise correctly. Purchase a book that contains workout plans as well as illustrations on correct form.
- Hire a personal trainer for a couple of sessions to orient you to proper form and use of equipment.
- Most personal trainers offer group-training sessions at reduced prices.
- Hire a personal trainer to work with you and a friend. It will keep down the cost, be motivational and fun.

- You don't need a gym to get in a good workout. I have worked out for years in my home with just a few inexpensive pieces of equipment, such as a jump rope, a couple of dumbbells, resistance bands, and a yoga ball.
- Work out at home with video CD's or DVD's, or your favorite TV exercise personality. I am a big fan of in-home workouts. A couple of my favorites are P90X and Insanity by Beachbody. These are intense workouts not meant for everybody. If you are more of a beginner or looking for less intense workouts try yoga or Pilates. The point is to do what you can at home or at a gym.

> You don't need a gym to get in a good workout. I have worked out for years in my home with just a few inexpensive pieces of equipment, such as a jump rope, a couple of dumbbells, resistance bands, and a yoga ball.

I can't afford fitness equipment.

- If you really can't afford any equipment, there are exercises you can do without any equipment at all. Start by walking or running.
- Get creative, use the world around you as your gym. Climb stairs, do pushups, use a retaining wall to do step ups. Go to the park and use the jungle gym or monkey bars.

I can't afford to eat healthy.

- You can't afford *not* to eat healthy. Fresh fruits and vegetables are the best foods you can put in your body.
- Preparing your own food at home not only is less expensive than eating out, you can control what goes into your meals.

Exercise is hard.

- Anything worth having is hard. Don't focus on the effort, focus on the results.
- You don't have to work out super hard for it to be effective.
- Easy exercise is better than no exercise at all.
- Wear a heart rate monitor to ensure you are working out at the right intensity and not overdoing it.
- The good news is, the more you exercise, the easier it gets.

I don't know how to begin.

- Visit your doctor for clearance before you begin any exercise routine.
- Learn as much as you can. Read books and articles, talk to friends who exercise, hire a personal trainer, go see a nutritionist.
- Go online for support. There are plenty of websites with information on how to begin an exercise regimen. Google it.

I don't know anything about nutrition.

- Good nutrition is not complicated. Go online for information on good healthy eating habits.
- Follow some simple guidelines for eating right. Reduce processed foods and sugars. Aim for a diet that consists of 40 percent carbohydrates, 30 percent fat and 30 percent protein. Eat lean proteins and whole grains along with plenty of fruits and vegetables.
- Reduce your portion size.
- Improve your knowledge of nutrition by reading the nutritional information provided on the labels of the foods you buy.

I'm too old.

- You're never too old to start living a healthier lifestyle.
- See your physician before embarking upon a new exercise program.

- Start slowly and gradually increase the length and intensity of your workouts.

You're never too old to start living a healthier lifestyle.

- It's a myth that as we get older, we naturally get larger. For most, it is a function of lifestyle, not age.

I'm afraid to fail.

- The only real failure is to not start at all. What have you got to lose?
- You haven't failed until you've given up.
- There are plenty of sources of support available to keep you from feeling like you've failed.
- Better to have failed trying than to never have tried at all.
- There's always tomorrow. Get back up on that horse. Yesterday is in the rear view mirror. Keep looking forward.
- Losing weight, maintaining fitness and eating healthy are not one-time events. There's always right now to start fresh.
- Keep a positive attitude and stay committed.
- Surround yourself with people who will support you when you're feeling down or unmotivated.

You haven't failed until you've given up.

I'll start tomorrow.

- Be honest with yourself, will you really start tomorrow? How many times have you told yourself that before?
- Why wait until tomorrow? If you wait until tomorrow, chances are there will be more weight to lose than if you start today.
- Sounds like an excuse not to get going today. Where is the excuse coming from? Why not today?

I can't get motivated.

- Sometimes we are just not in enough pain to feel the motivation. Special K, a popular cereal brand has a slogan, "How much will you gain when you lose?" I love that saying. Focus on the results and you'll find your motivation.
- Set clear and attainable goals. Put together an attainable plan and execute it. These are the keys to motivation.
- Find support if you need it. Friends, co-workers, even online forums are good sources of support to help you through moments when you lack motivation.

> Focus on the results and you'll find your motivation.

Let's face it, excuses are a way of life, but we don't have to let them prevent us from having the fit and healthy life we want to lead. No matter what your circumstances, you can lose weight, eat right and get or stay fit by changing just some of your lifestyle habits.

For many people, making excuses not to exercise or eat right is their greatest barrier to weight loss and fitness success. Don't let that be you. Stop the excuses and create healthy and positive habits that help you along your way to becoming a healthier, happier you.

CHAPTER 5 EXERCISES

What is it worth to you to accomplish your goals and dreams?

_____

_____

_____

_____

What is it costing you to stay stuck?

_____

_____

_____

_____

What is it going to take for you to change?

_____

_____

_____

_____

What do you want more: to change or to stay stuck?

_____

_____

_____

_____

What are your excuses?

_____

_____

_____

_____

How will you overcome them?

_____

_____

_____

_____

What will your life be like when you reach your goals? Envision it and write it down.

_____

_____

_____

_____

You can find these and all the exercise templates on our website at http:// www.slimpreneur.com/resources

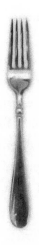

CHAPTER 6:

Barriers to Success

You may have to fight a battle more than once to win it.
—Margaret Thatcher

Your Beliefs Determine Who You Are

Countless barriers to success seem to be all around us. Most likely, the biggest barrier to our success is us. We create our success and we limit it as well. Often our belief system gets in our way. We determine who we are by what we believe.

We all have thousands of beliefs that affect us each and every day. Our beliefs are both positive and negative and they effect our perceptions and our actions. If we act positively and believe negatively we are on the road to disaster.

Our beliefs are not as abstract at you might think. Your beliefs determine what you do on a day-by-day basis. Your beliefs about your self-worth determine your wealth. Your beliefs about your health and fitness determine what you look like.

Let's say for example that you are ordering a meal at a restaurant. You decide to order food that is aligned with your beliefs about what is healthy and nutritious. The result of that decision will determine how you feel the rest of the day. Will you feel energized and fully functional? Over the course of time, your small decisions add up and determine your appearance as well as your overall fitness. Staying true to your beliefs about your health and fitness will determine your actions and affect how you look and how you feel.

Over the course of time, your small decisions add up and determine your appearance as well as your overall fitness. Staying true to your beliefs about your health and fitness will determine your actions and affect how you look and how you feel.

Can your current beliefs get you to the destination that you desire or are they holding you back? Beliefs are created over time and if we fail to challenge them, we are condemned to repeating our same old actions. Many of the beliefs you are holding now are holding you back and preventing you from getting to where you want to go.

Consider the story of a young girl who grew up overweight. People made fun of her. When she tried to do anything athletic she felt inadequate and stopped. She grew up believing that she could never be a runner, or cyclist or look great in a bathing suit. For a long time she never challenged those beliefs, and her life was okay, but not the life she dreamed of. She stayed inactive and no one pushed her to change.

One day she decided to challenge those beliefs. She got sick and tired of being sick and tired. She started exercising, just a little at first and on her own so she wouldn't be ridiculed. As she gained more confidence she joined a gym. Slowly her self-perception changed and she started to challenge herself athletically. Her body started to change and her self-confidence grew.

Today she's capable of anything she puts her mind to and her life is limitless. That girl is me.

Like me, most people come to a point in their lives when they realize they don't have to follow their old patterns and beliefs. That moment is powerful and liberating, but also can be frightening—a little like jumping off a cliff hoping there's a safety net. You're the only one who can make that decision. It's your choice: you can remain stagnant in your old beliefs or you can take a risk and move forward in your life. The choice is yours. You determine your beliefs.

Consciously choosing what to believe is powerful. Making your own choices as to what your beliefs are give them much more weight and meaning. I decided to intentionally throw away all those beliefs about what I couldn't do physically, what I couldn't look like and trusted my own new beliefs about what I wanted to become.

Like me, most people come to a point in their lives when they realize they don't have to follow their old patterns and beliefs. That moment is powerful and liberating, but also can be frightening—a little like jumping off a cliff hoping there's a safety net.

I realized, with the help of coaches and mentors, that for anything in my life to change, I had to change my thinking. Change had to come from the inside out, not the outside in. Is this your moment to challenge your beliefs and get what you really want?

Telling Yourself You Can't

Telling ourselves "we can't" is a common practice and one that often times we do unconsciously. We don't even realize we are doing it. I remember signing up for my first big bike ride. I'll admit I had doubts I'd be able to finish. During many of those training rides I recall facing a steep hill saying to myself, "I can't make it." I could have stopped and gotten off the bike and walked, but I didn't. I put the bike in a low gear and I pedaled. As I pedaled, I used to count down from 10 to 1, one count for each pedal stroke. Then I'd repeat that, over and over again until I reached the top. Baby steps, but I never gave in to the "I can't make it" in my head. By the time my first 100-mile bike ride came along I *chose* to make it and I did.

It is important to keep in mind that beliefs are neither good nor bad, they just are. The key is to *identify* your beliefs and make a conscious decision to keep the ones that serve you and jettison the ones that don't. You get to choose.

Telling yourself you can't is a cop out. I'm sorry but I just don't buy the "I can't" excuse. Don't get me wrong, I understand priorities and "I can't" may very well mean, "I can't right now," but I'll challenge that excuse as well. "I can't" often means "I don't want to," "I don't want to work that hard," or more likely, "I'm afraid to try; what if I fail?" These all are excuses that will result in you staying stuck, right where you are.

> Beliefs are neither good nor bad, they just are. The key is to *identify* your beliefs and make a conscious decision to keep the ones that serve you and jettison the ones that don't. You get to choose.

People who change their lives don't use that kind of language. They don't use those words. Successful people, be it in business or health and fitness say "I will" "I'll give it everything I've got," and "I'll commit." Successful people challenge their thinking, change their thinking and take decisive action. What actions will you take today to move you closer to having the health and fitness life you desire?

We all have limiting beliefs; it's what we do with them that counts. To escape their limits, follow these four steps to change them: Identify them, challenge them, replace them, and then take action.

The first step is to identify them. Begin to be conscious of the thoughts and beliefs that come up for you when you attempt something outside your comfort zone. Pay particular attention to the negative or limiting beliefs. It may be helpful to trace those beliefs back to where they originated. What we heard about ourselves growing up shapes what we believe as adults. Our parents, siblings, friends, family, and others all influence our thoughts about ourselves, which leads to our beliefs. As a result, we end up believing certain things about ourselves that hold us back.

Once you've identified those limiting beliefs, challenge them. Are they really true? Is it really true that you can't? Probably not. Challenge and then replace the limiting thought with a positive one. Then take action. Nothing is more empowering than taking positive action towards achieving what you want.

Limiting beliefs are powerful in that they tend to keep showing up in all facets of our lives. If your limiting belief is that you are not good enough, or don't deserve success, those thoughts will hold you back in everything that you do. If your underlying limiting belief is that you don't deserve to be fit and beautiful and healthy, guess what? You may have some success in that area, but eventually you will fulfill your underlying belief that you don't deserve it and you'll fall short of your goal, or have difficulty maintaining it. When you recognize your limiting beliefs, only then can you overcome them.

So how do you overcome your limiting beliefs once you've identified them? As I've said before, change comes from the inside out. You have to change what you believe. It's easier than it sounds.

There are numerous ways to change your programming, from psychotherapy to neuro-linguistic programming to a whole host of other complicated and expensive techniques. I personally subscribe to a simple yet effective method; bombard your subconscious.

There are many ways to access your subconscious mind: reading, listening, touching, and seeing are all ways of creating an electrical impulse that creates a connection that gets reinforced in the brain. To recondition your old programming, you must overwhelm your subconscious mind with positive programming in the form of declarations and positive affirmations.

As Loral Langemeier says in her New York Times best-selling book, *Yes! Energy: The Equation to Do Less, Make More*, "Those who commit to Yes! Energy lead their lives from a core knowing of calm, relaying a positive energy and optimism that is contagious and life affirming to those around them."

The first step is to create your new positive affirmations. Affirmations should be short statements that reinforce positive beliefs. Affirmations should be positive. Negating ones like "I won't eat that chocolate cake" or "I won't miss a workout" do not work because your subconscious mind glosses over the "not." Instead, it focuses on eating chocolate cake or missing a workout.

Affirmations should be written in the present tense, as if they already are true.

Affirmations should be written in the present tense, as if they already are true. Your unconscious mind does not know the difference between the past and the present and will take whatever you think literally. If you say, "I will be fit, healthy and weigh 130 pounds," your subconscious will take that to mean it will happen some time in the future. Instead, state your affirmative belief in the present tense: "I am fit, healthy and a beautiful 130 pounds."

By creating positive affirmations and reading, writing, seeing and hearing them over and over again, they become positive thoughts that erase your negative limiting beliefs. Once you've created these positive thoughts and ingrained them into the unconscious part of the brain, they work twenty-four hours a day, seven days a week on your behalf to create the life you want.

Another way to create affirmations and new beliefs is to make an audio recording of yourself talking about your new beliefs, and then listen to it several times a day. If you want to change your beliefs about your health and fitness, describe your life as a result of adopting your new beliefs. Describe everything as if it is already happening. Create a script and record it with music in the background. Listen to the recording during your workouts.

The way to measure the results is to keep taking action—keep doing the things outside your comfort zone that will move you toward your goal. As your beliefs change, your comfort zone expands to include them. Keep taking those actions that move you closer to your health and fitness goals—they'll not only get easier; you may even start to enjoy them!

The Dreaded Plateau

You're following your plan, eating right and exercising, and for weeks the weight is slowly coming off. Then all of a sudden, seemingly out of the blue—the scale won't budge. You are doing the exact same things, but they stop working. You've hit the plateau.

First, I want to let you know that almost everyone has experienced the plateau and has felt your frustration. Plateaus are a normal part of the weight loss journey, so know you are not alone. I know plateaus are maddening, but we all have them. Just remember the key is that small changes can make big differences. Changing your workout schedule, activity and intensity level can help you break through the plateau.

 Changing your workout schedule, activity and intensity level can help you break through the plateau.

Reasons You Stop Losing Weight

Reason 1: Weight loss plateaus are as predictable as they are explainable. Your BMR–basal metabolic rate–is defined as the energy your body needs to keep your body functioning at rest. It is the minimum amount of calories your body requires to do the most basic of functions. BMR accounts for approximately 60 to 70 percent of the calories you burn and is dependent on a person's body mass. As you lose weight your body mass shrinks. A good thing for sure, but as your body mass gets smaller, so does your BMR or number of calories needed to sustain your body.

For example, you weigh 165 pounds and you eat 2000 calories a day. You cut your intake by 600 calories a day and the weight starts dropping off. For a while, you lose weight eating 1400 calories a day. However, at some point you lose enough weight to decrease your BMR. This means that your body no longer burns 1400 calories per day; instead, at your new lower weight, it only burns 1100 calories. Plus, because there's less of you to move around, you're burning fewer calories when you exercise too. Welcome to the plateau.

Reason 2: Your body gets used to the increased level of exercise. As you do an exercise over and over, your body gets more efficient at performing that motion, and your body burns fewer calories doing it. For example, the first time you get on the treadmill you may be huffing and puffing and barely able to endure ten minutes. Weeks later, you're breezing through a forty-five minute workout. Your muscles learn how to move in such a way as to create the least amount of resistance.

This ability for the body to adapt is innate and would be vital if you were fighting for your very survival. However, when your goal is to burn as many calories as possible, it's not so desirable. Whether your body is getting used to resistance training with weights, running on a treadmill, or cycling three times a week, physical adaption is one of the most common reasons for a plateau.

Reason 3: You're stressed out. There is some truth to the excuse, "I didn't gain weight; I'm just retaining water!" Both physical and emotional stress can lead to fluid retention, commonly referred to as water weight gain. Technically speaking, stress resulting in an increase in the hormone estrogen, a decrease in progesterone or testosterone or an overstimulation of the adrenal glands can lead to fluid retention.

Reason 4: Lack of sleep. Studies have shown that lack of sleep can result in a plateau of weight loss or actual weight gain.

Reason 5: Your diet may be to blame. It's common to underestimate the calories you eat. Sometimes portion sizes creep up. Look for places where calories hide: condiments, dressings, sauces, and dips. Are you snacking between meals, tasting while preparing meals, or finishing food off your kid's plates? Could alcohol be to blame? Are you sneaking just a taste of dessert?

Strategies for Getting Off the Plateau

Put that frustrating plateau in your rear-view mirror with these proven strategies.

Strategy 1: Change it up. Increasing physical activity or just changing the exercises you do can lift you off the plateau. If you are doing cardio, add resistance training. If you are doing resistance training, add cardio. Add interval training to your routine. Interval training involves short bursts of high-intensity work integrated into your regular workout. For example, if you usually do steady-state workouts on the elliptical trainer, try two to five minutes of regular effort, then one minute of all-out effort and repeat. Strive for four to eight high-intensity intervals per workout.

Increasing intensity and adding resistance or weight training increases muscle mass which leads to a higher BMR, which means your body burns more calories. More muscle mass also burns calories for a longer period of time after your workout.

 Change it up. Increasing physical activity or just changing the exercises you do can lift you off the plateau.

Strategy 2: Avoid getting bored. Boredom is one of the most common reasons people stop exercising. At first, be sure to choose exercises you enjoy doing. Move outdoors if you're tired of the same four walls at home or at the gym. Try new exercises. If your gym has organized classes, try something new like Tae Bo or Zumba. Work out with a friend or hire a personal trainer. Mix up your weight training with thirty- to sixty-

second bursts of cardio between sets. Increase the amount of weight you lift or number of reps. Learn new weight lifting exercises. Keep your body guessing and yourself motivated by changing your routine once a month.

Strategy 3: Slow down. Sometimes backing off training and concentrating on eating right will nudge you off your plateau. This may sound counter-intuitive, but an over-trained, stressed body can hoard fat and stop weight loss. Be sure you avoid excessive training and adequately recover, which may require additional amounts of the right kind of calories.

Strategy 4: Keep a food journal. Write down everything you eat. Often over time we lose the edge and extra calories creep into our diet. Keeping track of everything that you eat will help you identify where the problem areas may be. Track the time of day that you eat and how you feel when you eat, if you think that emotional eating may be the culprit. Online and smart phone applications for food journaling make it easy to stay on track. A couple of my favorites can be found at www.livestrong.com and www.loseit.com.

Strategy 5: Cut your calorie intake by 100 to 200 calories a day. Here are some suggestions on how:

- Increase protein at breakfast which will help reduce calories consumed at lunch
- Substitute low- or non-fat cheese
- Eat a piece of fresh fruit instead of cookies or chips
- Substitute whole grains
- Try fat free ice cream or sherbet instead of regular
- Make your sandwich "open-faced" by eliminating one slice of bread
- Eat heart-healthy dark chocolate and cut down on portion size

Pay attention to how hungry you are.

Cutting your daily consumption by just a small amount may move you beyond your weight loss plateau.

Strategy 6: Take care when dining out because you're giving that restaurant kitchen control of what goes into your meal and how much shows up on your plate. Once it gets in front of you, you'll be tempted to eat every bite, right? Always approach a meal out with a strategy so you don't get caught off guard. Pay attention to how hungry you are. There is no rule that says you have to order an entrée. Order an appetizer or a salad instead of a main dish. Share an entrée or determine before you eat that you will bring half home in a doggie bag. Don't be afraid to make special requests. I often ask for a chicken breast with steamed vegetables. I always ask for the dressing on the side. If possible, limit dining out to special occasions and always have a plan in mind.

 Always approach a meal out with a strategy so you don't get caught off guard.

Strategy 7: Eat more protein. Some research shows that eating more protein can lower hunger. Protein works by suppressing ghrelin, a hormone secreted by the stomach that stimulates hunger. Studies have shown that fat and carbohydrates increase the level of ghrelin, thus causing an increase in hunger. Eating protein lowers levels of ghrelin substantially reducing the feelings of hunger. Take care not to overdo it though; protein should not exceed 30 percent of your daily calorie intake.

Strategy 8: Eat more fruits and vegetables. This one may seem like a no-brainer but warrants being repeated. Fruits and vegetables fill you up while providing much needed fiber and nutrients. Eating lots of low-calorie, high-volume fruits and vegetables makes you feel full and prevents you from eating more high-calorie and high-fat foods. Pile your plate with lots of vegetables and eat them first. Start out your meal with a salad, (light on the dressing), or a bowl of broth based vegetable soup. Stock your kitchen and refrigerator with lots of fresh fruits and vegetables and be sure to include them in every meal. Doing so will boost your intake of healthy vitamins, minerals, antioxidants, phytochemicals and fiber. Filling up on fresh fruits and vegetables will make it less likely you'll reach for high-calorie, processed snacks.

Strategy 9: Reconnect with your drive. If your motivation and drive is waning or you are feeling deprived, get back in touch with why you began down this path in the first place. Write down all the reasons you originally wanted to and still want to lose weight. If you've created your affirmations, get back into the practice of repeating them several times a day. If you've fallen off the wagon a few times or suffered a setback, forget it. Tomorrow is another day. Get back up on the horse and ride!

The Role of Aging in Weight Gain

The sad truth of the matter is that as women age, most tend to gain weight. They say these excess pounds are "normal," but they are not inevitable. Some say that an expanding waistline is the price of getting older, but I've seen some middle-aged women with smokin' bodies so I'm not taking the middle-aged spread lying down. Literally!

Studies reveal what we're up against. Statistically, the most significant weight gain in a woman's life tends to happen in the few years leading up to menopause called perimenopause. During this time and after the onset of menopause, body fat in women tends to shift from the arms, legs and hips towards the abdomen, where most of us call it belly fat. It is also true that each decade your metabolism slows down by ten percent and you lose eight percent of your muscle mass. All the more reason to focus on physical fitness and keeping fit, regardless of your age.

As you age, your lean-muscle mass generally diminishes and fat accounts for a larger percentage of your body weight. Lower muscle mass also results in fewer calories burned, which can lead to weight gain. Middle-aged women are most likely to see this weight gain as belly fat, due to a decreasing level of estrogen, which plays a part in where fat resides in the body.

While hormones do play a part in middle-age weight gain, it is not the only contributing factor. Eating habits and lifestyle changes can play a role as well.

Studies have shown that menopausal women tend to exercise less than other women. That fact, when combined with losses in lean-muscle mass that reduce the number of calories burned, can lead to weight gain. Genetic factors can also play a role. If your parents or close relatives tend to carry extra weight around their abdomen, chances are you're likely to do the same. Living a more sedentary lifestyle has also been found to contribute to weight gain.

Research indicates that this increase in belly fat not only makes it difficult to fit into your skinny jeans, it also can pose some health risks. Weight gain after menopause increases the risk of high cholesterol, high blood pressure and Type 2 diabetes. These conditions in turn increase the risk of serious diseases such as cardiovascular disease, stroke, breast cancer, and colorectal cancer.

That's the bad news. Here's the good news: preventing weight gain after menopause is not always easy, but it is simple. Once again, the choice is yours.

Preventing weight gain after menopause is not always easy, but it is simple. Once again, the choice is yours.

Strategies to Avoid Middle-Age Spread

While there is no secret formula, the strategies are the same basic ones we've been discussing so far.

Get up and move. A combination of aerobic activity and strength training is best for shedding those extra pounds or preventing them in the first place. We know that increased muscle mass helps burn more calories, so don't neglect muscle-building exercises. The Department of Health and Human Services recommends moderate aerobic exercise for at last 150 minutes a week or vigorous aerobic activity for at least 75 minutes a week. They also recommend strength training at least twice a week.

Watch what you eat. To maintain your current weight, you need about 200 fewer calories a day in your 50's than you needed in your 30's and

40's. Eat plenty of fruits and vegetables, lean protein and whole grains. Limit your intake of saturated fat, found in meat and high-fat dairy such as cheese and butter. Watch your intake of refined sugars, processed foods and sodium. Avoid prepared foods and fast food. Prepare your own meals whenever possible.

Keep portion sizes in check. In this day of supersizing meals it's easy to overeat even if you are making healthy choices. At home watch your portion sizes and avoid excessive snacking. When dining out, ask for the meal prepared without sauces, creams or oils. Order an appetizer instead of an entrée. Share an entrée or pack up half in a doggie bag before you begin eating.

Demand support. Surround yourself with friends and family who support you in your efforts to eat a healthy diet and encourage you to stay active. Instead of a lunch or dinner at a restaurant with a friend, suggest a hike or brisk walk followed by a healthy snack. Try something new like a yoga or Pilates class. Create a support group at work or with friends and meet once a week to exchange experiences, challenges, recipes, ideas and celebrate your successes. The bottom-line? Don't take getting older and getting fatter lying down. It's your life, go out and live it!

CHAPTER 6 EXERCISES ✐

What are your limiting beliefs?

_____

_____

_____

_____

What do you tell yourself you cannot do?

_____

_____

_____

_____

Write down your positive affirmations.

_____

_____

_____

_____

What are your strategies for getting up off the plateau?

_____

_____

_____

_____

You can find these and all the exercise templates on our website at http://www.slimpreneur.com/resources

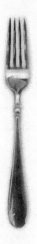

CHAPTER 7:

Tools for Lifelong Change

Do. Or not do. There is no try.
—**Yoda,** *The Empire Strikes Back*

For many the easy part of getting healthy is losing the weight; the hard part is keeping it off. I can relate to that. I lost and gained weight over and over until I finally discovered what worked for me. I'll share my strategies with you, but first, let's hear from the experts.

What the Experts Say

The National Weight Control Registry (NWCR) studied close to 3,000 people who had lost over 30 pounds and kept it off for over a year. Regardless of how the weight was lost, be it sensible or fad dieting, their study focused solely on how to keep the weight off. What they found was, although people lost the weight differently, the ways they kept it off were similar. What their study found was that to some degree, maintaining weight loss includes some common factors. These factors include:

- Eat a low-fat diet, but not a restrictive one.
- Watch portion size.
- Eat breakfast every day. Four out of five of those studied ate breakfast every day.
- Keep physically active. The most common form of exercise for those studied was walking, which they did for at least an hour a day.
- They found pleasure in their healthier lifestyle and felt liberated from constant dieting.

Overwhelmingly the participants who maintained their weight loss found that it got easier over time. They discovered what worked for them and what didn't. They stuck with the things that worked, which in turn gave them a feeling of satisfaction knowing they could stay in control.

I've seen it first hand in my clients, my friends and in myself. Energized about losing weight, you stick with the program and the weight comes off. Once you reach your weight loss goal, you go into maintenance mode. This is where the real challenge begins. You're good for a while, maybe even a long time, but eventually you slip back into old habits. Keeping the weight off in my opinion is harder than losing the weight in the first place. While I whole-heartedly agree to guidelines resulting from the study above, I'd like to share with you some of my personal strategies for keeping the weight off, as well as some I've learned from friends and clients.

> Once you reach your weight loss goal, you go into maintenance mode. This is where the real challenge begins.

Strategies for Keeping the Weight Off

Weigh yourself once a week. I intentionally listed this one first. I believe it is one of the best ways to keep on track. We talked about avoidance behaviors in Chapter 5, and this is a huge one. The scale doesn't lie. Keeping track of your weight every week lets you stay in control and aware of subtle changes, i.e. weight gain that you may not notice in the way your clothes feel until it's out of control.

Keep a food journal. When I was losing weight, my food journal was my best friend. Like the scale, the food journal doesn't lie and kept me on track and aware of what I was eating. It not only kept me up to date on how many calories I was consuming, but also revealed whether my diet was well balanced. My journal not only tracked calories, but fat, carbohydrates and protein. It was an easy way to ensure I had the nutrition I needed. My journal also kept track of my exercise and calories burned, which came in handy when I hit a plateau and used it to discover that I wasn't eating enough calories to fuel my workouts.

When I was losing weight, my food journal was my best friend.

Once I lost the weight, I eventually stopped using my food journal and started slipping back into some of my old bad eating habits. I stopped watching my portion sizes and slowly started to gain some of the weight back. Today I'm back to keeping my food journal as an everyday practice, regardless of whether my goal is to reduce or maintain. Either way, I'm staying on track.

Eat lots of fruits and vegetables. Find the fruits and veggies that you love most and eat tons of them. I strive for at least one vegetable with every meal. My goal is to fill my plate with two-thirds vegetables and split the remainder between protein and whole grains. Often I skip the whole grains and just have a lean protein pared with steamed or sautéed vegetables. I always eat my vegetables first, which may seem odd to some, but has become second nature to me. Eating lots of fruits and vegetables ensures that I get all the nutrients I need.

Eat a balanced portion of protein with every meal. Protein fuels your body and your muscles for your workouts. Protein feeds your brain so you can think clearly. Protein keeps you feeling full from one meal to another.

I've always struggled to include enough protein in my diet until I discovered protein powder. Protein powder can be used in shakes, stirred into yogurt, sprinkled over oatmeal or just mixed with milk or water.

Don't skip meals. Skipping a meal slows your rate of metabolism and may cause your body to store fat. Skipping meals may also lead to overeating later in the day. My recommendation is to eat three moderately sized meals and two small snacks throughout the day. This maintains a steady blood sugar level and prevents hunger that can lead to overeating or overindulging in the wrong kinds of foods.

Always eat breakfast. Studies have shown that you have a much greater chance of keeping the weight off if you start your day with a healthy breakfast.

Be prepared. Have you ever been out running errands or traveling for business and all of a sudden, you realize it's time for lunch or dinner and you're starving? Have you ever, at that decision point, chosen to visit a fast food joint even though you knew it didn't fit into your food plan? I know I have, until I learned to always be prepared. I always carry a back up with me. In my car I always have some kind of protein bar. I also carry one in my purse. If I know my day's schedule won't give me access to the foods I need to stay on track, I prepare my stash of travel foods. You will find a list of my travel foods in the Resources section in the back of the book or on our website, http://www.slimpreneur.com/resources.

Keep exercising. Studies show that physical activity is the single biggest predictor of long-term weight loss. Maintain a combination of aerobic activity and strength training.

Beware of self-induced inhibitors. A national survey by the Calorie Control Council found that 41 percent of women blamed weight gain on a lack

> Have you ever been caught hungry and chosen to visit a fast food joint, even though you knew it didn't fit into your food plan? I have— until I learned to always be prepared.

of self-discipline, while 36 percent stated they ate for emotional reasons. Determine what your triggers are, identify them and always be on the lookout for them. If your weak point is self-discipline, use a food journal to keep you honest. Stop looking at weight loss as a hardship and revel in the new healthier, thinner you. Find foods that keep you feeling satisfied instead of deprived. If emotional eating is an issue for you, recognize your triggers and be prepared. Have healthy alternative foods on hand, but limit yourself to small portions. Discover alternative outlets for your stress: take a walk or a run, meditate, or take a couple of deep breaths. Identify the source of your emotions and deal with them without turning to food for comfort.

Reward yourself–my personal favorite. As if losing weight and keeping it off isn't reward enough, I like to take it up a notch by occasionally splurging on me. I love jewelry, so twice a year if I've kept the weight off, I go buy myself something sparkling. Nothing expensive—just a reminder that congratulates me for a job well done. The point is to reward yourself with non-food pleasures you enjoy, like a massage, a manicure, or a new dress. For every goal you meet, you deserve a reward.

> Reward yourself with non-food pleasures you enjoy, like a massage, a manicure, or a new dress. For every goal you meet, you deserve a reward.

Share with friends. I have several friends who either want to lose weight or maintain weight they've lost. We have our own support group in which we share our ups and our downs. We hold each other accountable; we trade funny stories; we admit our shortcomings, share our challenges, and celebrate our successes. You don't have to do it alone; that wouldn't be half as much fun!

Weight Loss Maintenance — It's All in Your Head

While following a set of strategies to maintain weight loss is extremely important, part of keeping the weight off is the mental component, or what goes on in your head. Establishing the right habits and maintaining them is a basic key to weight loss maintenance.

It used to be said that you could form a habit by repeating an action for twenty-one days. New research suggests that it takes considerably longer: sixty-six days to form a new habit. Either way, once a habit is fixed in your subconscious, it is on autopilot, guiding you and your actions.

Establishing good habits depends on changing your beliefs on the inside. Through repetitive positive thoughts, affirmations and actions, you can establish new beliefs and thus form new habits that result in sustained weight loss maintenance. Failing to do so is the reason people frequently gain the weight back. They use determination and will power to starve themselves and lose weight, but don't change the programming and self-image that made them eat the way they did and gain the weight in the first place. Don't let this be you!

CHAPTER 7 EXERCISES

What are your strategies for lifelong change?

_____

_____

_____

_____

_____

What are your strategies for keeping the weight off or staying fit?

_____

_____

_____

_____

You can find these and all the exercise templates on our website at http:// www.slimpreneur.com/resources

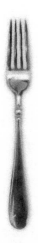

CHAPTER 8:

Changing the Way You Think Will Change the Way You Look

The first problem for all of us, men and women, is not to learn, but to unlearn.
—Gloria Steinem

Change from the Inside Out

Maxwell Maltz, in his long-time bestselling book *Psycho-Cybernetics* introduced the idea that a person must have an accurate view of his- or herself before setting goals. Otherwise, he or she would remain stuck in a pattern of limiting beliefs. Cybernetics refers to the control-and-response systems found in machines and animals that work much like a thermostat or missile guidance system.

Imagine you were on a plane that has charted a course to your destination. If while on the flight the pilot turns the plane twenty degrees to the right, you'll find the plane "rights" itself and shifts back to the original course. This is because there is a cybernetic mechanism on the plane that sends a signal to an automatic response system to return the plane to the programmed course whenever there is a deviation from the set plan.

Your brain also has a cybernetic mechanism. This explains why people who win the lottery spend all the money, and why people who lose weight gain it all back again.

Your past conditioning has resulted in your expectations. To achieve lasting change you have to rewrite your program. Willpower and determination will not work. You have to reprogram your brain before you get the results you want. You have to change from the inside out. As you grow and move to the next level of your life—be it achieving your weight-loss goals, improving your level of fitness, or success in your business—you will experience fear, doubt and anxiety.

> Highly successful people have all the same feelings of doubt and anxiety; it's how they react to them is different.

This is normal. Highly successful people have all the same feelings of doubt and anxiety; it's how they react to them that is different. Successful people, when faced with doubt, fear or failure, don't take it personally. They stand up to it and try something different.

The Laws of the Universe

The Universe is the most perfect and orderly of states. It is in perfect equilibrium at all times, and yet we take it for granted. We take for granted nature, the planet earth, our bodies, everything around us. Each is perfection governed by precise laws.

Once you understand these laws and how they affect your life, you can use them every day to work from a higher order of vibration. You'll understand how to guide your mind and your body to do what they need to do to manifest your goals and desires.

These laws are based on research from quantum physics and studies on the brain only recently discovered over the last decade. These laws relate directly to your life and they are irrefutable. Understanding them and how to use them will change your life.

I first learned about these laws of the Universe from Bob Proctor and subsequently dove deeper through the works of John Assaraf. Both have shown me how understanding of the laws of the Universe lets me get out of my own way, get in sync

These laws relate directly to your life and they are irrefutable. Understanding them and how to use them will change your life.

with the power of the Universe, and achieve my dreams and desires. My hope is that you too will use these universal laws to achieve your hopes and dreams, in all areas of your life.

The One Great Law—Energy Is.

There are seven natural laws of the Universe. Each of these falls under one over-arching law: *Everything is energy.* Everything you see, touch or is, is made up of energy. Even inanimate objects like the book you're reading right now is made up of energy. Everything is made up of, receives and emits energy. The following seven corollaries tell us how energy operates in the natural world and in our everyday lives.

Law One: The Law of Vibration and Attraction

Everything in the Universe constantly vibrates and moves. The difference between things we can see and cannot see is the frequency of the vibration. Thoughts, which we cannot see, are made up of energy and have a level of vibration. Negative thoughts like "I feel fat" produce negative vibrations, which then align you with other negative vibrations resulting in negative outcomes. Like attracts like. Your negative vibration attracts other people with similar energy and the results will be you will get the result you asked for: you will be fat. As Eckhart Tolle asks in *The Power of Now,* "Do you realize that the energy you thus emanate is so harmful in its effects that you are in fact contaminating yourself as well as those around you?"

It's up to you to decide whether you feel good or bad—and whether your vibration is high or low—by choosing your thoughts. Your willingness to choose positive thoughts ultimately results in getting what you want on the physical plane.

Law Two: The Law of Polarity

Everything in the Universe has an equal and exact opposite. This is also known as the law of yin and yang. If there exists something that is hot, there exists a polar opposite that, by law, must be equally cold.

Remembering this law can change the way we think and the way we react to challenges. The sooner we begin to look for opportunities instead of staying mired in our challenges, the sooner the negative disappears from our perception. Our energy changes and we get what we want.

> Recognizing and embracing the positive in every situation moves you closer to realizing your dreams.

Every situation has its silver lining, even the most difficult of circumstances. Recognizing and embracing the positive in every situation moves you closer to realizing your dreams.

Law Three: The Law of Rhythm

Everything is moving in perfect rhythm and at perfect speed. If you've ever been caught in the ocean's undertow and successfully navigated your way out of it, you know that fighting the current is futile. Swimming across the current, rather than against it is the way out. No matter how strong a swimmer you are, fighting will leave you exhausted, if you're even able to get out. Not fighting for your life is counter intuitive until you learn that going *with* the flow, rather than against it, can save your life. The ocean can teach us much about the rhythm of life. You live in a current when you resist the natural rhythm of life. Learn to recognize when you are out of sync with the current of the Universe. Stay focused on your dreams and go with the flow instead of fighting against it.

Law Four: The Law of Relativity

Everything is relative. If I asked whether you are tall or short, you couldn't really answer without comparing your height to something else. It is really up to your perceptions to define how you see things. The reality is that things just are.

Let's take a 35-foot yacht. To some people a boat that size is huge; to others who are used to a much larger ship, a boat that size is small. The reality is, the 35-foot yacht is neither large nor small: it just is.

This law teaches us that everything is relative and just is. While there may *seem* to be those who are more fortunate than we are, as well as those who are less fortunate, in reality things just are. As soon as we are able to look at situations in our lives without judgment of better or worse, we'll stop feeling like we're not enough or don't have enough.

Law Five: The Law of Cause and Effect

For every cause there is an effect, and for every effect there is a cause. According to the laws of physics, for every action, there is an equal and opposite reaction. This means everything you do causes an effect. If you think good thoughts, good thoughts come back to you. If you give love, you get love returned to you. The Universe will return to you what you put out there. Don't be stingy with your time, your money, your knowledge, or your gifts. Live life in abundance and you will receive abundance in return.

Law Six: Both Male and Female are Necessary for Creation

Many people think of this law as yin and yang, a perfect give and take, an exchange of energy that manifests in nature as male and female. Take the genderless context of a conversation between two people. The first person speaks, conveying an idea, thought or question while the other listens. Then roles reverse and the person who had been speaking listens. Out of this type of exchange, knowledge is transferred, new ideas explored, agreements are made. This give and take, yin and yang gives rise to new creation.

The law of gender manifests in all living things as masculine and feminine. In the example above, masculine energy is represented by the person speaking, while the feminine energy is represented by the listener. This law governs creation, and creation requires both masculine and feminine energy.

This law goes on to say that new creation comes from seedlings that require a gestation period. This is particularly true for thought seeds. Every idea has a gestation period; your job is to choose and cultivate the correct ideas and beliefs. Don't be in a hurry, let your new beliefs blossom in their own time.

Law Seven: Energy is Forever Moving Into and Out of Different Forms

Energy is everywhere, in constant flow from one form or vibration to another. This explains why the energy you surround yourself with comes back to you. If you surround yourself with negative thinking people, that is the energy that will flow back to you. It is true that the thoughts you have dictate the results you see. Your negative thoughts have energy and that energy flows to everything that surrounds you. Likewise, positive thinking has energy that flows in and out of all that is around you. You get to choose, surround yourself with positive or negative energy? It all starts with you.

These are the laws of nature and they are irrefutable. They are also meaningless unless you get off the couch and get into action. You must do something every single day that propels you towards your goals. Being in action and staying in action is the key to your success.

However, it is not all about being in action. Our society teaches us to be "doers" with messages like, "Go, go, go," "Always be in action," and "Stay on the treadmill of life and you will find success." We have not been taught much about "being." How can we get out of the rat race and begin to work in harmonious vibration with the world around us, the way the Universe works?

The third law of the Universe, the Law of Rhythm, provides the answer: the least amount of effort always wins over the greatest amount of effort. If you find that you are stressed out and pushing back, it's because you are not working with the laws of the Universe. The Universe looks for the easiest, fastest way to accomplish its goals, and you should too!

CHAPTER 8 EXERCISES 🖋

How has your past conditioning contributed to your current results?

_____

_____

_____

_____

Choose one of your negative or limiting thoughts and re-program it into a positive thought.

_____

_____

_____

_____

Write down three ways you are fighting life. Re-program them into positive, go-with-the-flow energy.

_____

_____

_____

_____

Get into action. Write down the actions you will take today.

_____

_____

_____

_____

_____

_____

You can find these and all the exercise templates on our website at http:// www.slimpreneur.com/resources

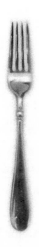

CHAPTER 9:

Commitment and Accountability

We are what we repeatedly do. Excellence, then is not an act, but a habit.
—**Aristotle**

The January Syndrome

It's a Monday morning in late January, and I'm feeling fat. The holidays are long over and reflecting back on the season, I'm really angry with myself. I can identify two things that happened since Thanksgiving: I let myself go and paid little attention to my usual healthy eating plan, and I slacked off and paid little attention to work because it was the holiday. Don't get me wrong—enjoying the holiday is okay, even encouraged—and I did it intentionally, knowing that come January, I'd put my head down and get back to work. So here I sit, Monday morning after a Sunday full of football, beer and fattening snacks, facing February 1, and I'm still in holiday mode.

So Monday morning I vow to get back on track, to deprive myself, to work out until it hurts, and—guess what? I'm back on the merry-go-round. If this sounds like you, you're not alone. You and I are not the only ones to put control on hold during the holidays. Unfortunately that means many of us start the year with an extra five to ten pounds. We're already behind in our health and fitness goals and the year has just begun. We feel the pressure to catch up.

We also feel the pressure to catch up with work after enjoying some well-deserved time off. For many of us the holidays are a slow time in our business anyway, so we take it a little easier. Then January comes and BAM! We're "back to it," often feeling we need to make up for lost time. We focus on working more and that's always a good excuse for neglecting our health.

Well, no more. The secret to getting off that bandwagon is never again to put yourself in the situation where you feel that way. Take back control of your life! I love the holidays and I do expect to eat a little more, drink a little more and maybe not work out as much, but you don't gain weight after a day or two of splurging. You gain weight when you tell yourself, "I'll eat now and get back to my regular routine later..." days later, weeks later, or even a month later.

The key to keeping on track is to never let yourself get too far off track.

The key to keeping on track is to never let yourself get too far off track. Easier said than done I know, but keeping your weight loss and fitness goals in the front of your mind each and every day is the key. Take a day off here and there, and splurge on your favorite foods once in a while. There's nothing wrong with a holiday celebration as long as you treat each day as an opportunity to start over, eat right, and exercise more.

Whatever you do, don't throw your hands up and say, "I give up. It's too hard. I'll get back to it later." After a particularly challenging situation where you didn't keep to your goals, don't dwell on it! Tomorrow is another day. Get back on track tomorrow. A day or two of falling off the wagon will not amount to weight gain

Always treat each day as an opportunity to start over, eat right, and exercise more.

or a loss in fitness. Be good to yourself, stop beating yourself up and take back your control. That in itself will give you the strength to push forward and succeed.

Taking time off work to spend with family and friends is a very good thing, but doing so adds pressure come January to make up for lost time and productivity. For many of us who are entrepreneurs, we are the business and if we're not there, business grinds to a halt. You know what? That's okay. Build the time off in to the business plan. That way you will be free to not only enjoy yourself during the holiday, but you can reenter the New Year free of guilt and stress.

In my business, the holidays are a slow time. People are busy and many put coaching on the back burner as they spend time with their loved ones. I like to use the time between Christmas and New Year's to clean my office, tie up loose ends for the year ending, and put together my goals for the coming year. I find that focusing on my goals for the coming year helps me stay on track during the holidays because my goals are in the forefront of my mind. I also use the holiday time to reflect on the past year, which helps me identify what is working and what is not working; as well as ways to make the coming year more productive and successful. I honor what I accomplished in the current year, and use any

I firmly believe that things happen as they are supposed to happen. When life throws you a challenge, it's your responsibility to figure out why you've been presented with it; what you can learn from it; and how it can make you a better person.

disappointments as a vehicle to learn why I failed to achieve a goal and how I can do things better.

I firmly believe that things happen as they are supposed to happen. When life throws you a challenge, it's your responsibility to figure out why you've been presented with it; what you can learn from it; and how it can make you a better person.

Are you familiar with the two-by-four rule? You see, life throws us little challenges. If we recognize them, determine what the lesson is, and learn that lesson, then life is good. But if we ignore the challenge or don't learn why we were presented with it, we get a more difficult challenge the next time: something a little bigger and a little more challenging to get our attention. If we continue to ignore these ever-more serious challenges, the Universe ultimately hits us across the forehead with a two-by-four, figuratively of course. Wham! Now that will get your attention. Look for the lessons in the small challenges before they grow to the point that they really hurt.

I do not make New Year's resolutions. I don't believe in them. However, I do believe in setting goals. I create SMART goals that help me stay focused on what is important and what I want to achieve in the coming year.

Setbacks are a part of life. We all have them. Anyone who has stretched to reach a goal that challenges them to work hard has experienced setbacks. It's just the way it is. I'd even go so far as to say that these experiences are what makes us strong and teaches us valuable lessons. It's not always easy to believe that in the moment however.

Interested or Committed?

I've always been an exerciser. I grew up in a family where my Dad was a runner, my Mother was an avid golfer, my brother was a natural athlete, and then there was my sister and I. Neither of us got much of the athlete gene, but both of us have worked out for as long as I can remember and continue to do so today. As a child, I was overweight, but as a young adult I found that exercise was my friend.

Most of what I did for exercise was in the gym and 90 percent of it was some kind of cardio. You could say I was a cardio junkie. For many years, my favorite workouts were high-intensity step aerobics, kickboxing or Tae Bo. In the winter of 2003, after what my sports medicine doctor told me was too much high-intensity aerobics, I found myself with not one, but two torn Achilles tendons. Dr. Looslie, a wise man who over the years had treated me for miscellaneous sports-related injuries, knew that a prescription of rest was not going to cut it with me. He recommended low-intensity stationary biking until my injuries healed.

For weeks I sat on that stationary bike, going nowhere, getting my legs back in shape. As I healed I began taking spin classes at my gym. Don't be fooled, they are quite a workout with the right instructor. I bought a bike and joined a group of female beginner riders who were training for an all-women sixty-mile bike ride that spring.

I fell in love with cycling. I joined a cycling club in the area, and even though I was always at the back of the pack, every weekend I was out riding. I did my first century (100-mile bike ride) that summer, and in July of 2005 I completed the Death Ride, one of the country's most difficult bike rides. I was 46 years old. I did the Death Ride again the next year at age 47. I completed my first triathlon at the age of 51.

I am not an athlete; I'm an exerciser. I've never been particularly athletic, I'm not that coordinated and I don't have any extraordinary skills. I'm an exerciser who is determined, loves a challenge, finishes what she starts and does what she says she'll do. I'm an exerciser who will not let my age or my weight, or anyone tell me I can't do something. We determine who and what we are, we determine what we can accomplish. It is completely up to us.

I trained for the Death Ride for six months. I hired a coach and did everything she told me to do. Everything. The day of the ride I was ready. My favorite

I am not an athlete; I'm an exerciser.

moment of that entire day came on the third mountain pass. I began the climb with my dear friend Dave, who had been my companion on hundreds of training rides. He was fast; I was not. He was always in the front and not once in all the rides we had shared had I *ever* beaten him to the top of a climb.

As we began the climb up that third pass, he said to me, "When I get to the top, I'll wait fifteen minutes and if you're not there by then, I'm taking off and I'll see you at the finish." I said okay and started my slow and steady climb. I passed him within the first hundred yards of the climb and never looked back. I beat him to the top of that mountain pass and waited there with the biggest Cheshire cat grin on my face you've ever seen. What made the difference? Training, determination, doing what you say you're going to do, and being accountable.

I beat him to the top of that mountain pass and waited there with the biggest Cheshire cat grin on my face you've ever seen.

What are you willing to challenge yourself to become right now? Whatever it is for you, you must be willing to push yourself to be more than you are right now. Whatever it is that you determine you want—be it weight loss, physical fitness, to finish a 5K run or marathon, whatever your goal may be—your success depends on three things and only three things: knowing where you are now, knowing where you want to go, and taking action every day to get there.

If you really want a better life than you have right now, do whatever it takes. If not, give yourself and those around you a break and just admit you're not willing to pay the price to have it all. Continue to whine and complain rather then get out of your comfort zone and do what's required to have a better life. Or choose to commit. Once you do, you'll find the process is easier than you could have ever imagined.

If you are truly committed, the process will be easy. A good friend of mine and fellow coach has a saying: *"Are you interested or committed?"*

Interested is fine and dandy, but if you really want change you must be committed. Committed means doing everything you possibly can, even when—and especially when—it's out of your comfort zone. Choose today to commit. Stay committed and you'll experience overwhelming success.

Are you interested or committed? Choose to commit. Once you do, you'll find the process is easier than you could have ever imagined.

The Energy of Commitment

People who achieve success—whether with weight loss, fitness, their business or in their relationships—know what they want and through their actions, they achieve it. Often times they achieve more than they ever thought they could. Successful people define their goals, work and train, fall down and get back up again until they get what they want. I recently heard a motivational speaker say that the more you fail, the more successful you become. I believe that if you learn from every one of those failures, every one of them makes you stronger.

Be willing to commit to realizing your dreams. Expand your mind to imagine yourself better than you are right now, more fit, more healthy and energetic. Find someone who believes in you more than you believe in yourself. Find someone

People who achieve success — whether with weight loss, fitness, their business or in their relationships — know what they want and through their actions, they achieve it.

who has walked the path you are embarking on and has been successful. You don't have to do it alone.

It's a funny thing about commitment: once you do it, things somehow have the tendency to fall into place. Any goal you have in life, any change you want in your life, has to start from the inside out. That may seem counter-intuitive to you or against what you've been taught, but the truth is our lives are ruled by certain laws of the Universe. We can understand and work with these laws or we can push against them and make our lives hard. Once we understand that everything in our lives is at this moment as it should be, and that we have the power to change our lives through our actions, our lives will start to change. The first step is always to commit. I like to talk about it as the Universe giving you what you want, once you are clear what that is and make a commitment to get it.

> Once we understand that everything in our lives is at this moment as it should be, and that we have the power to change our lives through our actions, our lives will start to change.

The next step is to get into action, positive action. I believe everything is made up of and emits energy. We emit and attract energy every day, and the type of energy that flows around us is determined by our energy. I've been told that a person's net worth can be determined by the average net worth of their ten closest friends. Meaning, like attracts like so the energy we send out is reflected in those around us and gets returned to us.

Jack Canfield, creator of the *Chicken Soup for the Soul* series, developed a three-part strategy for tapping into positive energy.

Step 1: Identify what you really want and eliminate the negative.

Focus on what you want rather than what you don't want. State your intentions and desires in positive words, eliminating negative words like "don't," "not," and "no."

Step 2 – Raise your vibration level.

Imagine how you would feel if you already had the things you want. Identify the things that make you feel good and do more of those things. Have zero tolerance for negative feelings. Raise your vibration level with positive affirmations. Raising your vibration level has everything to do with feelings and nothing to do with thinking.

Step 3 – Release it and allow it.

Release your affirmations, positive feelings and vibrations to the Universe and let go. The Universe will provide. Eliminate doubt.

Will Mattox is one of the most effective coaches I've ever worked with and he's been a great mentor to me. Long ago I hired Will to coach me. I knew I had much greater things inside of me and it was time for me to grow to the next level and stop playing small.

I had just quit my W2 job and was starting out as an entrepreneur. I knew I wanted to go into real estate development but had no idea what to do or how I would make money. On our first coaching call Will asked me how much money I wanted to make. I had been making $250,000 in my W2 job so I said "$250,000. Will said, "I don't think so, more." I said, "Okay, $300,000," to which Will replied, "More." I stammered, "$500,000??? I can't make $500,000 in a year!" Will said, "You're right. You can't make that much money because you just told me you can't." He gave me an exercise to spend fifteen minutes every day in the energy and belief that I could make $500,000 in a year.

On our next call, the first words I uttered were, "Guess what, Will—I'm going to make $500,000 this year." I believed it with every cell in my being. That year I exceeded that goal. Eliminate doubt and believe; the Universe will provide.

The Price of Success

Many people achieve financial success at the expense of the rest of their lives. They keep thinking that once they make a certain amount of money, then they'll finally have the time for other things like their health and fitness. Guess what—very few ever get there. There's always one more deal to make, just a little more money to be made and before they know it, it's too late. They have failed to realize that it's the journey, not the destination.

Many realize much too late that success really means finding fulfillment and balance in all areas of life.

> Many realize much too late that success really means finding fulfillment and balance in all areas of life.

We all know of people who sacrificed everything in pursuit of the almighty dollar only to die alone, or have a brush with illness that teaches them life is short. Life *is* short and we never know how much time we have left. Life is a series of tradeoffs that we make every day, every moment; we trade our lives for the actions we choose to take. Balance is the key to a successful life.

Many years ago I worked for a sales manager that actually told us that if we were in shape physically, we weren't working hard enough! Meaning, any time spent in the gym was time not spent in the office or on sales calls. I still shake my head at that today, but it did instill me with the belief that work took top priority, and that my fitness and health were a lower priority.

Over the years, I've come to know better. I know that if I don't have my health and can't work, who is going to do my work for me? I owe it to my family to be the best I can be and that starts with a strong body and mind. I wonder where all my fellow sales men and women are today. Are they overweight, lethargic and sick, or are they living the life of their dreams—healthy, wealthy and wise? Make the most of each day. Don't wait until "later" to have the balance you want in your life.

If you are a parent, you are aware that you are your child's most influential and significant role model. As that role model, it's your responsibility to teach your child what they'll never learn in school. Our school system teaches kids how to memorize facts and regurgitate them back. They don't learn how to think. They don't discover the answers to questions like, "Who can I become in my lifetime? How do I create a life of contribution and abundance? How do I become more so I can have more?" Most people play out their lives as they've been socially conditioned to do, without asking these empowering questions. Because our school system doesn't teach us to think, we need to revamp the system and give teachers the tools they need to properly condition our children to truly understand their capabilities and create high self-esteem.

You *can* have it all: health, fitness, great relationships and money. Stop just accepting that things are the way they are. Stop blaming your circumstances or the conditions to which you were born or brought up for your life today. *You* create your reality. The past is part of who you are. It helped shape you, but it does not limit who or what you can become. Almost every person I know who has experienced great success has overcome some level of adversity. By success, I mean fulfillment in all areas of their lives, not just one. The trick is to not allow the difficulties you encounter to define who you are, and more importantly, who you can become. Hard times craft who we become by challenging us to work through them and come out better on the other side.

Happiness is a choice, not a byproduct of our circumstances. You make the choice to be happy, or let the events and situations in your life weigh you down (pun intended). You may not like some of the things that happen in your life, but the choice to be

The trick is to not allow the difficulties you encounter to define who you are, and more importantly, who you can become.

happy about them is totally and completely yours. Once you accept the current circumstances of your life—such as that extra weight you're carrying and your current fitness level—it's up to you create a plan to better your life. You're creating your life every day anyway. Why not create the life of your dreams while you're at it?

CHAPTER 9 EXERCISES

Are you interested or committed?

_____

_____

_____

_____

What are you really willing to commit to, right here, right now?

_____

_____

_____

_____

Choose three of your SMART goals from Chapter 2 and write them down.

Goal One

_____

_____

_____

_____

Goal Two

_____

_____

_____

_____

Goal Three

_____

_____

_____

_____

What are your top three action steps for attaining each goal?

Goal One Action Steps

_____

_____

_____

_____

Goal Two Action Steps

_____

_____

_____

_____

Goal Three Action Steps

_____

_____

_____

_____

How or to whom will you be held accountable for achieving your goals?

_____

_____

_____

_____

You can find these and all the exercise templates on our website at http://www.slimpreneur.com/resources

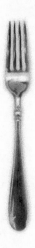

CHAPTER 10:

Don't Wait—Get Started Today

The future belongs to those who believe in the beauty of their dreams.
—Eleanor Roosevelt

You've explored current weight loss strategies and why they don't work. You've looked at yourself and others and identified methods of sabotage. You've looked at healthy eating habits and the role of exercise in weight loss and fitness. You've seen barriers to success, excuses and ways to get up off the plateau. You've seen how the way you think effects the way you look. Lastly, you understand the importance of commitment and accountability. Now it's time to pull it all together into your action plan. New ideas and strategies are great, but nothing changes until you get into action.

Start today! If you take away only one thing from reading this book, please let it be that each day is a new day, and that *you* control your destiny. Every day is a new beginning and an opportunity to change. Never beat yourself up for anything you've done or haven't done in the past. Take hold of your future and demand the life you deserve.

If you did not complete the exercises as you read through the chapters, go back and do so now. The exercises are designed to provide you with a starting point for your plan. You can find all the exercise templates on our website at http://www.slimpreneur.com/resources.

If you take away only one thing from reading this book, please let it be that each day is a new day, and that *you* control your destiny.

Your Next Step

Realizing weight loss and fitness success is a process. That process begins with you. Through the course of this book you have identified your goals and found sources of guidance and support as you move along your journey. The next step is to put what you've learned into action. So what does that look like?

We see success as a four-step process;

Step One – The first step towards achieving real success is to change what you're doing today - change your habits. Choose a time frame, we like 28 days or a month for instance, and change one thing you do or think about each and every day. What a great way to begin to really see how your thoughts, actions and behaviors effect the way you look and feel. We provide 28 days of actionable strategies to get you started toward your weight loss and fitness goals.

After 28 days you will experience subtle changes in the way you look, feel and think. Now it's time to really accelerate your progress.

Step Two is where you dig in and make things happen. In step one you took the first actions towards weight loss and fitness. Now it's time to kick your progress into high gear. Step two is a 90-day commitment to your success. Our 90-day program will have you making a serious commitment to getting what you say you want. Our workbook is like having your own personal coach in a box, guiding you through the various stages of weight loss and fitness; goal setting, defining you're motivation, recognizing self doubt, healthy eating habits, healthy exercise habits, avoiding excuses, getting inside your head, tools for lifelong change and maintenance.

You'll notice these are the very topics we've covered in this book. The difference with the 90-day program is that you'll not only be reading about them, you'll put them into practice. 90 days of actionable steps that you commit to and record in your workbook.

Step 3 is the accountability stage. We all need accountability. It is the key to success and without it we often fail to achieve our goals. Have you ever said you were going to do something and didn't do it? And nobody was the wiser? Nobody knew so the not doing got easier. Without someone to hold us to our word, we often fail to get what we really want because it's so much easier just not to do the work. Being held responsible for doing what we commit to is sometimes hard, but it's often the only way to get things done. Accountability looks like weekly, bi-weekly or monthly calls; group or one on one coaching to keep you on track.

Once you've reached your goals, the challenge is to maintain; weight loss, fitness, strength, whatever it is for you. **Step four** is all about staying motivated over the long haul. Strategies, support, forums, informational exchange, it's all about a focus on your individual needs to stay on track and maintain.

How Do I Get Started?

Right now, go to http://www.slimpreneut.com/freevideo and learn how you can begin, this very minute to change your habits and finally have the weight loss and fitness success you've dreamed about. It's our gift to you. Do it now. There's no better time to begin than NOW!

Resources

Online Tools

http://www.livestrong.com

http://www.loseit.com

http://www.weightwatchers.com

BMI Chart

For more information visit http://www.bmi-calculator.net/

Body Mass Index Table

Body Weight (pounds)

BMI	Normal						Overweight					Obese										Extreme Obesity															
Height (inches)	19	20	21	22	23	24	25	26	27	28	29	30	31	32	33	34	35	36	37	38	39	40	41	42	43	44	45	46	47	48	49	50	51	52	53	54
58	91	96	100	105	110	115	119	124	129	134	138	143	148	153	158	162	167	172	177	181	186	191	196	201	205	210	215	220	224	229	234	239	244	248	253	258
59	94	99	104	109	114	119	124	128	133	138	143	148	153	158	163	168	173	178	183	188	193	198	203	208	212	217	222	227	232	237	242	247	252	257	262	267
60	97	102	107	112	118	123	128	133	138	143	148	153	158	163	168	174	179	184	189	194	199	204	209	215	220	225	230	235	240	245	250	255	261	266	271	276
61	100	106	111	116	122	127	132	137	143	148	153	158	164	169	174	180	185	190	195	201	206	211	217	222	227	232	238	243	248	254	259	264	269	275	280	285
62	104	109	115	120	126	131	136	142	147	153	158	164	169	175	180	186	191	196	202	207	213	218	224	229	235	240	246	251	256	262	267	273	278	284	289	295
63	107	113	118	124	130	135	141	146	152	158	163	169	175	180	186	191	197	203	208	214	220	225	231	237	242	248	254	259	265	270	278	282	287	293	299	304
64	110	116	122	128	134	140	145	151	157	163	169	174	180	186	192	197	204	209	215	221	227	232	238	244	250	256	262	267	273	279	285	291	296	302	308	314
65	114	120	126	132	138	144	150	156	162	168	174	180	186	192	198	204	210	216	222	228	234	240	246	252	258	264	270	276	282	288	294	300	306	312	318	324
66	118	124	130	136	142	148	155	161	167	173	179	186	192	198	204	210	216	223	229	235	241	247	253	260	266	272	278	284	291	297	303	309	315	322	328	334
67	121	127	134	140	146	153	159	166	172	178	185	191	198	204	211	217	223	230	236	242	249	255	261	268	274	280	287	293	299	306	312	319	325	331	338	344
68	125	131	138	144	151	158	164	171	177	184	190	197	203	210	216	223	230	236	243	249	256	262	269	276	282	289	295	302	308	315	322	328	335	341	348	354
69	128	135	142	149	155	162	169	176	182	189	196	203	209	216	223	230	236	243	250	257	263	270	277	284	291	297	304	311	318	324	331	338	345	351	358	365
70	132	139	146	153	160	167	174	181	188	195	202	209	216	222	229	236	243	250	257	264	271	278	285	292	299	306	313	320	327	334	341	348	355	362	369	376
71	136	143	150	157	165	172	179	186	193	200	208	215	222	229	236	243	250	257	265	272	279	286	293	301	308	315	322	329	338	343	351	358	365	372	379	386
72	140	147	154	162	169	177	184	191	199	206	213	221	228	235	242	250	258	265	272	279	287	294	302	309	316	324	331	338	346	353	361	368	375	383	390	397
73	144	151	159	166	174	182	189	197	204	212	219	227	235	242	250	257	265	272	280	288	295	302	310	318	325	333	340	348	355	363	371	378	386	393	401	408
74	148	155	163	171	179	186	194	202	210	218	225	233	241	249	256	264	272	280	287	295	303	311	319	326	334	342	350	358	365	373	381	389	396	404	412	420
75	152	160	168	176	184	192	200	208	216	224	232	240	248	256	264	272	279	287	295	303	311	319	327	335	343	351	359	367	375	383	391	399	407	415	423	431
76	156	164	172	180	189	197	205	213	221	230	238	246	254	263	271	279	287	295	304	312	320	328	336	344	353	361	369	377	385	394	402	410	418	426	435	443

Source: Adapted from Clinical Guidelines on the Identification, Evaluation, and Treatment of Overweight and Obesity in Adults: The Evidence Report.

SlimPreneur
Fitness Test / Assessment

Name_____

Date _____

Before starting any new fitness routine, it is recommended that you visit
your doctor or health care professional to make sure you are ready to begin
an exercise regimen.

Once you've got the all-clear, take our health and fitness assessment. It
will help you identify exactly where you are right now. Our assessment will
help you determine where you want to be, and once you get there, you'll
never go back. Knowing how far you've come will provide much appreciated
motivation once you've achieved your goals.

Take "before" photos to chronicle your progress.

Perform body fat analysis. There are several methods to determine your
body fat percentage: DEXA scans, hydrostatic weighing, measurement with
calipers or use a scale that has BIA, bio-electric impedance analysis that
measures how much of your body is water and how much is fat.

Body Fat Percentage: _____

Body Fat Recommendations:

	Fit	Athlete	Elite Athlete
Men	14 to 17%	10 to 13%	4 to 9%
Women	21 to 24%	16 to 20%	12 to 15%

Take your measurements:

Weight	_____	Right Thigh	_____
Chest/Bust	_____		Left Thigh _____
Waist	_____	Right Arm	_____
Hips	_____	Left Arm	_____

This is a series of exercises designed to gauge your general fitness level and act as a benchmark for your progress.

Resting Heart Rate Test

Start by taking your resting heart rate. If you have a heart rate monitor, use it! Relax for 2 minutes before taking your resting heart rate. If you don't have a heart rate monitor, take your pulse from your wrist or neck, count your heart beats for 30 seconds, multiply by 2 to get your resting heart rate.

Resting Heart Rate _____

Step Test for Aerobic Fitness

Using a 12-inch step or the stairs in your home, step on and off for three minutes. Step up with your right foot, then your left foot, step down with your right foot, then your left. Continue with a steady and consistent pace, up, up, down, down for three minutes. Once complete, immediately check your heart rate. Check the table below to see how you compare to the average person of your age and gender.

Step Test Heart Rate _____

AVERAGE RESULTS FOR STEP TEST FITNESS

Male

Age	26 - 35	36 - 45	46 – 55	56 - 65
Excellent	<81	<83	<87	<86
Good	81 – 89	83 – 96	87 – 97	86 – 97
Above Avg	90 – 99	97 – 103	98 – 105	98 – 103
Average	100 – 107	104 – 112	106 – 116	104 – 112
Below Avg	108 – 117	113 – 119	117 – 122	113 – 120
Poor	118 – 128	120 – 130	123 – 132	121 – 129
Very Poor	>128	>130	>132	>129

Female

Age	26 - 35	36 - 45	46 – 55	56 - 65
Excellent	<88	<90	<94	<95
Good	88 – 99	90 – 102	94 – 104	95 – 104
Above Avg	100 – 111	103 – 110	105 – 115	105 – 112
Average	112 – 119	111 – 118	116 – 120	113 – 118
Below Avg	120 – 126	119 – 128	121 – 129	119 -128
Poor	127 – 138	129 – 140	130 – 135	129 – 139
Very Poor	>138	>140	>135	>139

Push-Ups: Upper Body Strength Test

This test determines how many push ups you can do in one minute. You should use the standard military-type push-up. Keep your back straight as you lower your chest to the ground. Feel free to do push-ups on your knees if you desire. Count the total number of push-ups you can do and record the amount below.

Number of Push-Ups _____

AVERAGE RESULTS FOR PUSH UP FITNESS TEST

Male

Age	26 - 35	36 - 45	46 – 55	56 - 65
Excellent	<47	<41	<34	<31
Good	39 – 47	34 – 41	29 – 34	25 – 30
Above Avg	30 – 38	25 – 33	21 – 28	18 – 24
Average	17 – 29	13 – 24	11 – 20	9 – 17
Below Avg	10 – 16	8 – 12	6 – 10	5 – 8
Poor	4 – 9	2 – 7	1 – 5	1 – 4
Very Poor	>4	>2	0	0

Female

Age	26 - 35	36 - 45	46 – 55	56 - 65
Excellent	<36	<37	<31	<25
Good	30 – 36	30 – 37	25 – 31	21 – 25
Above Avg	23 – 29	22 – 29	18 – 24	15 – 20
Average	12 – 22	10 – 21	8 – 17	7 – 14
Below Avg	7 – 11	5 – 9	4 – 7	2 – 6
Poor	2 – 6	1 – 4	1 – 3	1
Very Poor	0 – 1	0	0	0

Sit-Ups: Abdominal/Core Strength Test

This test determines how many sit ups you can do in one minute. Lie on your back on the floor with your knees bent, feet flat on the floor. Your hands can rest on your thighs, but do not grab your thighs to help you up. Sit up until your hands reach the top of your knees. Be sure to keep your lower back on the ground as you come up. Never arch your back or let your lower back leave the floor! Do not pull yourself up with your hands behind your neck or head. Count the total number of sit-ups you can do in a minute and record the amount below.

Number of Sit-Ups _____

AVERAGE RESULTS FOR SIT UP FITNESS TEST

Male

Age	26 - 35	36 - 45	46 – 55	56 - 65
Excellent	<45	<41	<35	>31
Good	40 – 45	35 – 41	29 – 35	25 – 31
Above Avg	35 – 39	30 – 34	25 – 28	21 – 24
Average	31 – 34	27 – 29	22 – 24	17 – 20
Below Avg	29 – 30	23 – 26	18 – 21	13 – 16
Poor	22 – 28	17 – 22	13 --17	9 --12
Very Poor	>22	>17	>13	>9

Female

Age	26 - 35	36 - 45	46 – 55	56 - 65
Excellent	<39	<33	<27	<24
Good	33 – 39	27 – 33	22 – 27	18 – 24
Above Avg	29 – 32	23 - 26	18 – 21	13 – 17
Average	25 – 28	19 - 22	14 – 17	10 – 12
Below Avg	21 – 24	15 - 18	10 – 13	7 – 9
Poor	13 – 20	7 --14	5 -- 9	3 – 6
Very Poor	>13	>7	>5	>3

Wall Sit: Lower Body Strength Test

We're going to test your lower body strength by seeing how long you can hold a wall sit. Place your back flat against a wall and lower yourself until you are seated with your legs at a 90-degree angle. Begin timing and hold the position as long as you can without affecting your form. Place your hands on your thighs, legs together. As soon as you start to come out of the 90-degree position, stop timing. 30 seconds is average. 60 seconds is good, 90 seconds is excellent.

Wall Sit _____ seconds

Record all your data at the beginning of your fitness program. Choose an amount of time and retest. I suggest you repeat the fitness test every 30 days to track your progress.

Good luck on your fitness goals. We're here to support you in your fitness journey. Feel free to contact us if you have any questions. http://www.slimpreneur.com/contact-us/.

Travel Strength Training Workout

One of the biggest challenges many of us have is how to keep up our workout routines while on the road. While many of the hotels I've stayed at recently have fitness facilities on site, some charge a fee, (the last hotel I stayed at charged me $15 per day to use their workout room) while some don't have any place to work out at all. While running outside is sometimes an option, not all of us love to run and sometimes the weather can be uncooperative. Finding a workout routine that is suitable to do in a hotel room and is challenging enough to make us feel like we've gotten a good work out would be the ticket to staying on track on our fitness and weight loss goals.

I have found that a resistance band workout is great for when I'm traveling. The bands fit into my suitcase without taking up much room and I can work out in my hotel room or outside, whichever is more convenient.

Exercise bands are readily available at most sporting goods retailers. For best results, purchase a set of bands with various levels of resistance to maximize your workouts.

Below are just a few of my favorite routines that I use on the road.

Band Workout for Travel

Stretching a band once may seem easy, but when you repeat the same move over and over (repetitions or "reps"), you feel the challenge building.

In this workout you're going to focus on the legs and the arms first, then the core and abs. You're going to do one leg exercise, one arm exercise, a second leg exercise, a second arm exercise, then repeat the whole sequence three times.

There is a good reason to alternate arms and legs. When you do one set of leg exercises, the blood rushes to your lower body as you complete the work. When you follow that immediately with an arm exercise, your body gets the message, "Hey, I need blood up here." This confuses the body, causing it to constantly react to your muscles' needs. This makes the body stronger and more efficient.

You'll finish strong with a set of abdominal exercises and a cool-down stretch.

THE WORKOUT

To warm up, do one of the following for 3 minutes

- March in place knees high
- Jog in place (optional, high impact)
- Jumping jacks (optional, higher impact)

Arms and Legs

Squats: 1 set of 8–12

Bicep Curls: 1 set of 8–12

Leg Side Raise: 1 set of 8–12 each side

Lateral Arm Raise: 1 set of 8–12

Wall Sit: 30 seconds to 1 minute

Repeat the Arms and Legs sequence two more times for a total of three sets for each exercise.

Ab/Core Workout

Core Leg Raises: 1 set of 8–12 reps

Straight-Legged Sit-Ups: 1 set of 8–12

Windmills: 1 set of 10 on each side

Repeat the Ab/Core sequence two more times for a total of three sets for each exercise.

Stretch

While on your back, turn onto your stomach, stretch your arms over your head. Reach your arms and legs as far in the opposite direction as you can, giving yourself a good stretch. Keep your head neutral. Take a couple of deep breaths, letting them out slowly.

Bring your hands under your shoulders, take a deep breath and push your torso upwards while exhaling. This is called a Cobra stretch. Keep your head high, stretch as tall as you can and hold for 10–15 seconds, taking deep breaths and letting them out slowly. Return to the mat or floor, then repeat.

Raise so that you are on your hands and knees, then sit back on your legs, and lower slowly into Child's pose. Legs are bent underneath you; your arms are reaching forward. Take a few more deep breaths.

Return to your hands and knees and stand up slowly, rounding your back up, feeling each vertebrae as you stand. Your head and arms should be the last things to come up. Raise your hands above your head and stretch.

Lower your arms and bend your right leg. Grab your toe and bend your leg so that your heel is close to your buttocks. Keep your knees together and hold the stretch. Feel free to hold onto wall or chair for support. Press your hip forward for a deeper stretch.

Repeat on the other side.

Round your shoulders forward, keeping your hands to your sides. Repeat for 6 shoulder rolls then change direction and roll your shoulders backwards for 6 reps.

Raise your hands over your head while taking a deep breath. Look to the sky, exhale and bend forward, with legs shoulder-width apart and touch your toes. Stand up slowly, rounding up, feeling each vertebrae as you stand. Repeat 2 more times, taking deep breaths.

Give yourself a hug and congratulate yourself for a job well done!

THE EXERCISES

Squats - Works your thighs and buttocks.

Stand with both feet on the band, shoulder-width apart. Raise your hands with the band handles to your shoulders, or higher until you feel a good resistance from the band. Squat as low as you can comfortably go, as if you were sitting on a chair. Hold for a second and stand up. Make sure your back remains flat, your head stays up and you're looking straight ahead. Never let your head drop or the shoulders round forward. Repeat for 8–12 reps.

Lateral Arm Raise - Works your shoulders.

Stand with both feet together on the band. Raise your arms out to the sides, hold for a second and lower. Repeat for 8–12 reps

Bicep Curls - Works your biceps.

Stand with both feet on the band, shoulder width apart. Start with your hands at your sides. Keeping your elbows close to your sides, raise hands to your shoulders, pause, then lower them to your sides. Repeat for 8–12 reps. You can alternate arms if you wish. You can also alternate bringing hands straight up for one rep and then slightly out to the side for the next rep.

Leg Side Raise - Works your outer thigh and hip.

Start by standing with both feet on the band. Pull the handles up towards your chest, keeping them close to your body. Standing on your left foot, raise your right foot out to the side as high as you can, keeping your leg straight. Pause for 1 second then lower. Repeat for 8–12 reps. Repeat on the left side.

Wall Sit - Works your legs and core.

Stand with your back up against a wall. Inch your legs out until you are in a seated position. Your legs should be at right angles to the floor. Hold for 30 seconds to 1 minute. For a greater challenge, go a few inches lower for the last 10–20 seconds.

Core Leg Raises - Works your legs and core.

Lay on your back on the floor or anywhere that is comfortable. Stretch your legs out, keeping your legs together and arms at your sides. Raise your feet to the ceiling, keeping your legs straight, till they are at a 90 degree angle. Flex your toes. Keep your lower back to the floor; do no let it raise off the floor. If you need some support, feel free to place your hands underneath your buttocks to keep your lower back from raising up. Lower your legs, keeping them as straight as possible until they almost reach the floor, but don't touch the floor. Pause for a second and raise your legs back to the ceiling. For a bigger challenge, use your band. Hold the handles and wrap the band under your feet. Pull on the band to create resistance while lowering your feet. Repeat for 8–12 reps.

Straight-Leg Sit-Ups - Works your abs and core.

Lay on the floor with your legs straight, spread apart at a comfortable distance. Sit up, raising your right hand straight up toward the ceiling, not in front of you, straight towards the sky. Stretch at the top, pause for a second, then bend forward, with your back straight (don't let your shoulders hunch over), and touch the opposite toe with the hand. Keep your head up and look forward. Sit up, then lay back down slowly, letting each back vertebrae touch the floor one by one. Repeat with the left side. Repeat for 8–12 reps per side.

Windmills - Works your abs and core.

Sit on the floor with your legs bent, leaning back slightly. Place your hands together in front of you. Turn to the right, keeping your hands together and touch the floor on your right side. Keep your back straight and sit tall as you twist. Return to the center. Twist to the left, keeping your hands together and touch the floor on your left side. If you want to challenge yourself, keep your feet together with knees bent and raise them a few inches off the ground. Repeat for 10 reps on each side.

To download a copy of this workout, please visit http://www.slimpreneur.com/resources.

Healthy Foods For Travel

I'm frequently asked, "What are the best foods to take with me when I travel?" I always carry healthy food choices with me. I like to be prepared and not leave what I eat up to chance or someone else's discretion.

The following is a list of the foods that I bring with me when I travel. I break them up by food that needs to be refrigerated and those that don't. These are just my suggestions and the foods I like. Be creative, have fun with it. I'd love to hear your suggestions of some of your favorite foods for travel.

Refrigerated Foods
- Hard Boiled Eggs
- Chicken Strips (Costco)
- Cheese/Mozzarella Sticks – Lite
- Carrot Sticks
- Yogurt: Fage 0 percent
- Yogurt: Low Fat or Non Fat, in individual containers
- Jicama
- Celery
- Skinny Cow Cheese Triangles
- Hard Cheese
- Cottage Cheese
- Salad

- Lettuce Wrap Sandwich
- Tortilla Wrap

Non-Refrigerated
- Turkey Jerkey
- Peanut Butter
- Dried Fruit such as raisins, craisins, mangos, apricots, cherries, and apples
- Oatmeal
- Apples
- Bananas
- Clementines
- Oranges
- Grapefruit
- Protein Shake Powder
- Power Bars or your choice of protein/energy bars
- Almonds or other healthy nuts
- Popcorn

Staples
- Green Tea
- Vitamins
- Crystal Light
- EmergenC

This list is constantly updated, to get the most recent version, please visit our website at:

http://www.slimpreneur.com/resources

Recipes

BREAKFAST

Almond Breakfast Bars   Serves 12

These yummy breakfast bars are great right out of the oven or wrap them up and take them with you on the road, to enjoy after your workout or on a hike.

1 cup applesauce

1 ¼ teaspoon ground cinnamon

2 cups bran flakes cereal

1 ½ cups Bisquick baking mix

¾ cups brown sugar

¼ cup butter, melted

1 egg or ¼ cup egg substitute

1 teaspoon vanilla extract

¼ cup almonds, chopped

Preheat oven to 350 degrees. Spray an 8 by 8 inch glass baking dish with nonstick cooking spray. Place the applesauce in a sauce pan and cook over medium heat. Cook until mixture is thick, stirring frequently, about 7 minutes. Remove from stove and stir in ¼ teaspoon of the cinnamon. Combine baking mix, cereal, brown sugar, butter and remaining cinnamon in a large bowl and combine until mixture resembles coarse crumbs. Stir in the egg and the vanilla and combine until mixture forms a ball. Press mixture into the bottom of prepared 8 by 8 inch pan. Cover with the applesauce mixture, spreading evenly. Sprinkle applesauce with the almonds. Bake for 30 to 40 minutes or until toothpick inserted into the middle comes out clean. Cool and cut into bars.

| Calories 226 | Fat 9.2g | Protein 6.5g | Carbs 34.1g | Sodium 71.4mg | Sugar 14.2g | Fiber 4.1g |

Kody Kakes   Serves 6

We love this healthy and nutritious updated version of the standard pancake. The bananas carmelize as they cook making these non-traditional pancakes sweet and delicious.

1 ½ cups Kodiak Pancake Mix

1 ½ cups water

1 medium banana, sliced

1 teaspoon cinnamon

Mix pancake mix with water until smooth with no lumps. Add the cinnamon. Pour ¼ cup batter onto skillet or pan coated with nonstick cooking spray. Immediately place sliced bananas on uncooked side of pancake. Turn pancakes when cooked and slightly brown. Cook another 3-5 minutes until cooked through. Serve.

Calories 116	Fat 0.75g	Protein 5.42g	Carbs 25.1g	Sodium 162mg	Sugar 5.0g	Fiber 3.7g

Greek Omelet

Serves 2

Easy to make with just a few garden fresh ingredients. Shake it up by adding fresh vegetables that you have on hand.

½ cup chopped tomato
2 tablespoons chopped scallion
3 kalamata olives, pitted and chopped
2 tablespoons chopped fresh basil
1 teaspoon balsamic vinegar
1 cup egg substitute
1 ounce feta cheese
salt and pepper to taste

Combine the first 4 ingredients in a small bowl. Lightly spray a nonstick skillet with nonstick spray. Heat skillet to medium heat and pour in the egg substitute. Cook until the underside starts to set, about 4 minutes. Sprinkle in the feta cheese and cook until cheese is just starting to melt. Spoon the tomato-olive mixture evenly onto the omelet. Once the omelet is cooked through fold over half of the omelet and cook one minute longer. Cut in half and serve.

Calories 157	Fat 5.9g	Protein 15.8g	Carbs 5.8g	Sodium 422mg	Sugar 4.6g	Fiber 0.87g

Fast Frittata Muffins   Serves 6

I like to make a batch of these and have them on hand for a quick and tasty breakfast on the go.

1 carton egg substitute, 16 ounce
¾ cup roasted red peppers in a jar
5 ounces feta cheese
1 package chopped frozen spinach, 10 ounce package
3 tablespoons skim or fat-free milk

Microwave spinach on high for two minutes to defrost. Wrap in a clean dish towel to drain excess liquid. Beat egg substitute and milk in a small bowl. Mix in feta cheese. Add chopped peppers, spinach and salt and pepper to taste. Pour into muffin tins coated with cooking spray. Bake at 350 degrees for 12 to 15 minutes, or until firm and just golden on top. Makes 12 muffins.

Once cooled, you can store the frittatas in the fridge. To reheat, microwave for 20 to 40 seconds, or pop them in a toaster oven for about a minute.

Calories 124	Fat 5.0g	Protein 14.9g	Carbs 5.0g	Sodium 458mg	Sugar 42.2g	Fiber 1.0g

Breakfast Protein Shake with Fruit Serves 1

I like to whip up this shake and take it with me when I'm on the go, to the gym or an early business meeting. This shake also makes a great mid-morning or afternoon snack.

2 scoops protein powder, 62 grams. I prefer Met-RX Protein Plus
1/3 cup strawberries
1/3 cup blueberries
1/3 cup blackberries

Mix all ingredients in a blender with 1 cup water or skim milk. You can add ice to your shake, but I prefer to freeze my fruit and add them frozen. Feel free to mix up your choice of fruit, add apples, blackberries, melon, bananas, pineapple, whatever is in season or you have on hand. Protein powder typically comes in chocolate and vanilla flavors. Either one works great for this recipe.

| Calories 281 | Fat 52.8 | Protein 46.7g | Carbs 22.9g | Sodium 127mg | Sugar 10.5g | Fiber 7.4 |

Veggie Egg White Omelet   Serves 2

Add any vegetables in season to spice it up. Make sure you get your daily allotment of fresh vegetables.

1 cup egg whites or 6 egg whites
½ red pepper, diced
¼ cup red onion, chopped
¼ cup shredded reduced-fat cheddar cheese

Sauté the peppers and onions over medium heat in a medium non-stick sauté pan, about 5 minutes until translucent. Add the egg whites and cook until almost set. Sprinkle the cheese over the egg whites and serve. Salt and pepper to taste.

Calories 113	Fat 2.6g	Protein 16.3g	Carbs 4.7g	Sodium 295mg	Sugar 0g	Fiber 1.3g

LUNCH

Smoky Butternut and Sun-Dried Tomato Soup   Serves 8

Smoked sun-dried tomatoes give this dish such an earthy and rich taste, you'd never guess it was low calorie. Creamy and delicious, it's great as either a side or main dish. Top with a dollop of non-fat sour cream for added richness. For a short cut, use a can of pureed butternut squash instead.

1 tablespoon olive oil
½ medium red onion, chopped
3 cups cubed butternut squash
4 cups chicken stock
1 28-ounce can crushed tomatoes
½ cup smoked sun-dried tomatoes
½ cup fresh basil or 1 ½ teaspoon dried
1 teaspoon red pepper flakes, optional
Salt and pepper to taste

Sauté onion and squash in olive oil in large stockpot on medium heat for 10 minutes or until softened, stirring frequently. If using canned squash, sauté onions and then add squash puree.

Add stock, sun-dried and crushed tomatoes; bring to a boil. Reduce heat and simmer, covered for 40 minutes.

Allow to cool slightly, transfer to a blender or use a hand blender and puree until smooth.

Return puree to pot; reheat to simmer. Add basil, salt and pepper to taste. Once heated through, serve with sprig of basil and dollop of non-fat sour cream.

Calories 111	Fat 2.9g	Protein 2.6g	Carbs 11.1g	Sodium 712mg	Sugar 6.4g	Fiber 3.6g

Vegetarian Stuffed Peppers   Serves 4

Red peppers make this dish sweet and colorful. Full of antioxidants, these stuffed peppers make great leftovers. We enjoy them in the summer, adding fresh vegetables in season. Kick up the heat by adding red pepper flakes or hot pepper sauce.

4 red bell peppers, halved, seeds removed
1 onion, chopped
2 garlic cloves, minced
1 can diced tomatoes, 14.5 ounce
1 can corn, drained, 14.5 ounce
1 can diced green chilies, 4 ounce
1 teaspoon chili powder
1 cup brown rice, cooked
½ cup reduced-fat cheddar cheese

Preheat your oven to 375 degrees. Bring a large pot of water to a boil, drop in the peppers and cook until just tender, about 5 minutes, then drain and cool.

Prepare the filling: Spray a nonstick medium pan with cooking spray and sauté the onions and garlic over medium heat until softened, about 5 minutes. Add the tomatoes, green chilies, chili powder, corn, and a dash of salt and pepper. Bring to a boil. Turn down to simmer and cook, stirring occasionally for 10 minutes. Remove from heat and stir in the rice.

Stuff each pepper half with the filling mixture and place in a 9 by 13 inch glass baking dish. Top with the cheese. Cover with foil and bake for about 20 to 25 minutes. Uncover and bake until the cheese melts and is golden brown.

Calories 249	Fat 3.4g	Protein 10.0g	Carbs 45.0g	Sodium 370mg	Sugar 10.2g	Fiber 6.2g

One Hundred Calorie Chili   Serves 16

This is one of my favorite staple dishes. It's quick to prepare, contains lots of healthy vegetables and is very versatile. Serve over a green salad for a wonderful Taco Salad.

½ pound ground turkey

1 onion, chopped

1 can black beans, drained, 14.5 ounce

1 can kidney beans, drained, 14.5 ounce

1 can non-fat refried beans, 14.5 ounce

1 can tomato sauce, 14.5 ounce

1 can diced tomatoes. 14.5 ounce

1 ½ cup water

1 package taco seasoning mix

1 can corn, drained

1 can green chilies, 4 ounce

2 yellow squash, diced

2 zucchini, diced

2 tablespoons chopped jalapeño, optional.

In a medium skillet, sauté and the onion and the ground turkey. Add all the remaining ingredients and heat until boiling. Reduce heat and simmer for 10 minutes. Serve. Optional toppings: reduced-fat cheddar cheese, non-fat sour cream, sliced scallions. Serving size – 1 cup.

Calories 107	Fat 2.7g	Protein 6.3g	Carbs 15.2g	Sodium 216mg	Sugar 1.7g	Fiber 3.2g

Teriyaki Meatball Salad   Serves 6

1 pound ground turkey
½ cup panko breadcrumbs
½ cup water chestnuts, chopped
  fine
½ cup teriyaki sauce
3 scallions, sliced fine
1 egg or equivalent egg substitute
⅓ cup rice wine vinegar
¼ cup olive oil
2 tablespoons light soy sauce

1 teaspoon sugar
Juice of 1 lemon
¼ teaspoon salt
¼ teaspoon pepper
½ teaspoon ground mustard
1 bag shredded coleslaw
1 cup shredded carrots
3 scallions, sliced
½ cup sliced water chestnuts

Preheat the oven to 400 degrees. In a medium bowl, combine ground turkey, panko, water chestnuts, 2 tablespoons teriyaki sauce, scallions and egg. Roll into 1-inch meat balls and place on a lightly greased baking sheet. Bake for 20 minutes or until cooked through. Toss with remaining teriyaki sauce.

To make the salad dressing combine vinegar, oil, soy sauce, sugar, lemon juice salt, pepper and mustard and shake to combine. To a large bowl, add one bag shredded coleslaw mix, carrots, scallions, and water chestnuts. Toss lightly with prepared dressing. Top with meatballs and additional sliced scallions.

Calories 343	Fat 7.0g	Protein 16.8g	Carbs 28.7g	Sodium 906mg	Sugar 14.7g	Fiber 2.9g

Open-faced Tuna Melt Sandwich   Serves 4

This is a twist on the usual tuna melt. Full of interesting flavors with a little crunch, you'll love this non-traditional addition to lunchtime.

4 slices sprouted wheat bread
1 can albacore solid white tuna, 7 ounce
1 tablespoon light mayonnaise
1 tablespoon Fage non-fat Greek yogurt
1 tablespoon sweet pickle relish
1 tablespoon red onion, chopped fine
1 tablespoon sliced jalapeño, chopped
4 slices reduced-fat pepper jack cheese

Drain the tuna. Mix it with mayonnaise, yogurt, relish, onions, and jalapeños. Spread ¼ of the mixture on each slice of bread. Top with cheese. Spray a non-stick skillet with cooking spray and cook open face sandwich till the cheese melts and the bottom is browned.

Calories 163	Fat 2.1g	Protein 14.6g	Carbs 18.9g	Sodium 445mg	Sugar 1.1g	Fiber 1.1g

Spicy Grilled Chicken Salad   Serves 4

Perfect for a warm summer evening, this refreshing salad can be eaten year round. This salad gets some heat from chili powder and cumin while keeping it's cool with mandarin oranges and water chestnuts. In a pinch add rotisserie chicken from the grocery store instead of grilling the chicken.

½ cup cilantro, chopped fine

Juice of one medium orange

¼ cup lime juice

2 shallots, finely chopped

2 garlic cloves, minced

1 teaspoon chili powder

1 teaspoon ground cumin

2 teaspoons honey

Four 3-ounce boneless skinless chicken breasts

8 cups romaine lettuce, torn

2 tablespoons olive oil

One 15-ounce can mandarin oranges

4 scallions chopped

One 8-ounce can sliced water chestnuts

Prepare the marinade and the salad dressing: in a small bowl combine the cilantro, orange and lime juice, shallots, garlic, chili powder, cumin and honey. Pour ½ cup into a gallon sized zip-lock bag, add the chicken and seal, squeezing out as much air as possible. Make sure the marinade coats all the chicken. Refrigerate at least 2 hours or overnight. Pour the rest of the dressing into a salad dressing container or jar, add 2 tablespoons olive oil and shake well. Keep refrigerated until needed.

Grill the chicken over medium heat until cooked through, about 35 minutes. Slice diagonally. To make the salad, combine the lettuce, mandarin oranges, scallions, and water chestnuts. Add the salad dressing; toss to coat. Top with sliced chicken. For added crunch add chopped cashews or peanuts.

Calories 256	Fat 3.1g	Protein 25.0g	Carbs 23.2g	Sodium 82mg	Sugar 13.7g	Fiber 6.2g

Thai Chicken Burrito   Serves 4

A great way to use leftover chicken or a rotisserie chicken, this burrito is light, yet satisfying.

2 teaspoons sesame oil
4 cups shredded coleslaw mix
4 scallions, sliced
2 cups rotisserie chicken or cooked chicken, cubed
4 tablespoons dry roasted peanuts
4 teaspoons lime juice
1 tablespoon light soy sauce
2 10-inch flour tortillas
4 tablespoons fresh cilantro, chopped
¼ teaspoon red pepper flakes, optional

Heat the sesame oil in a nonstick skillet over medium heat. Add the coleslaw mix, scallions and red pepper flakes to taste. Cook, stirring frequently until cabbage begins to wilt, about 4 minutes. Stir in the chicken, lime juice and soy sauce. Cook until heated through, about 3 minutes more. Remove from heat and stir in the peanuts and cilantro. Spoon half of the filling into each tortilla and roll up. Cut in half on a diagonal and serve.

Calories 310	Fat 19.1g	Protein 16.8g	Carbs 16.8g	Sodium 516mg	Sugar 3.5g	Fiber 2.0g

Asian Chicken Salad   Serves 4

4 boneless, skinless chicken breasts, 3 oz
1 teaspoon lime zest, grated
3 tablespoons fresh squeezed lime juice
1 tablespoon honey
1 tablespoon fresh ginger root, minced
3 tablespoons light soy sauce
1 tablespoon olive oil
1 head romaine lettuce, chopped
1 mango, chopped
1 red bell pepper, cut into strips
1 can sliced water chestnuts (6 oz)
½ cup fresh basil, chopped
2 scallions, sliced thin on diagonal
4 teaspoons toasted sesame seeds

Heat a large skillet to medium high heat. Season the chicken with salt and pepper. Add to pan and cook 6 minutes per side or until cooked through. Optionally grill chicken on BBQ for added flavor. Slice chicken and set aside. In a large bowl, whisk together the lime juice, zest, honey, ginger, soy sauce and oil. Season with a pinch of salt. Gently add the lettuce, mango, bell pepper, water chestnuts, and basil. Toss to combine. Place ¼ of the salad mixture on each plate, top with ¼ of the chicken. Sprinkle with sesame seeds and serve.

Calories 321	Fat 7.3g	Protein 29.5g	Carbs 16.6g	Sodium 226mg	Sugar 9.9	Fiber 3.2g

DINNER

Chicken Enchilada Stew   Serves 4

1 pound chicken breast, diced into 1-inch cubes
1 ½ cups Trader Joe's Enchilada Sauce
1 cup onions
1 tablespoon garlic
1 can diced green chilies, 6 ounce
1 can black beans, 12 ounce

Sauté onions, garlic and diced chicken breast over medium heat in a medium-sized sauce pan until brown. Add the remaining ingredients and simmer for 10 minutes on low heat. Serve.

Calories 201g	Fat 6.8g	Protein 22.1g	Carbs 14.7g	Sodium 928 mg	Sugar 4.4g	Fiber 2.5g

Spicy Turkey on Lettuce Leaves   Serves 6

2 ounces rice noodles

1 tablespoon dark sesame oil

2 teaspoons freshly grated ginger

3 cloves garlic, minced

1 pound ground turkey

½ cup red bell pepper, seeded, and finely chopped

1 carrot, finely chopped

1/3 cup cucumber, finely chopped

1/3 cup red onion, finely chopped

6 tablespoons rice vinegar

2 tablespoons honey

¼ cup light soy sauce

¼ cup cilantro, chopped fine

3 tablespoons dry roasted peanuts

12 lettuce leaves

garlic chili paste

Cook the rice noodles according to the directions on the package. Rinse under cold water and drain. Chop fine. Heat 1 teaspoon of the sesame oil in a non-stick skillet. Add the garlic and ginger and cook, stirring for about 30 seconds. Add the ground turkey and cook through. Transfer to a large bowl, adding the bell pepper, cucumber, carrots, onion and noodles.

In a small bowl combine the vinegar, honey, soy sauce, cilantro, peanuts and remaining sesame oil. Add garlic chili paste to taste. Add to the ground turkey mixture and toss well. Mound the turkey mixture into each lettuce leaf and serve.

Calories 273	Fat 15.7g	Protein 12.9g	Carbs 18.5g	Sodium 486mg	Sugar 8.3g	Fiber 1.7g

Lasagna Olé   Serves 8

A take on ordinary enchiladas, this dish resembles a Mexican lasagna. The dish can be prepared ahead of time and refrigerated until ready to bake.

2 teaspoons olive oil	2 cans chopped green chilies, 4.5
1 pound ground turkey	ounce
1 large onion	1 teaspoon red-wine vinegar
2 garlic cloves, minced	¼ cup fresh cilantro, chopped
1 teaspoon dried oregano	4 6-inch flour tortillas, halved
¼ teaspoon ground cumin	1 cup reduced-fat cheddar cheese,
2 bottles of enchilada sauce, 10	shredded
ounce	Salt and pepper to taste

Preheat oven to 375 degrees. Spray an 8.5 by 11 inch lasagna dish with cooking spray. In a large non-stick skillet, heat 1 teaspoon of the oil. Add the ground turkey, half of the onions, half of the garlic and a pinch of salt. Cook until browned. In a medium sauce pan over medium heat, add the remaining 1 teaspoon of oil. Add the remaining onions, garlic, oregano, cumin and a pinch of salt. Cook until vegetables are softened but not brown. Add the enchilada sauce, chilies and vinegar, bring to a boil. Reduce heat and simmer, covered for about 10 minutes until flavors have blended. Remove from heat and stir in the cilantro. To make the casserole, arrange 4 of the tortilla halves on the bottom of the lasagna dish. Spoon half of the turkey mixture over the top and add half of the sauce, cover with half of the cheese. Repeat, layering the tortillas, meat, sauce and cheese. Cover the dish loosely with foil, bake 20 minutes or until bubbly and heated through. Remove the foil and bake for an additional 5 minutes until cheese is brown and bubbly. Let stand 10 minutes before serving.

Calories 249	Fat 10.5g	Protein 19.3g	Carbs 20.0g	Sodium 541mg	Sugar 1.2g	Fiber 1.6g

Chipotle Pork Chops   Serves 4

This dish is great with pork chops or pork loin. Pair with Black Bean Salad found in the Sides section.

1 teaspoon ground chipotle chili powder
1 teaspoon paprika
1 teaspoon ground cumin
1 teaspoon ground coriander
1 tablespoon olive oil
4 pork chops or pork loin, 3 ounce
Salt and pepper to taste

Heat the oven to 375 degrees. In a small bowl, combine the chipotle, paprika, cumin, coriander and olive oil and pinch of salt and pepper. Stir until the spices form a paste. Coat the pork with the spice mixture. Bake on a baking sheet about 25 minutes, until cooked through and firm to the touch. Remove from the oven and let stand for 5 minutes before serving.

Calories 218	Fat 16.7g	Protein 15.9g	Carbs 0.9g	Sodium 1300mg	Sugar 0.1	Fiber 0.63g

JFish Fish Tacos   Serves 8

Super easy to put together, this dish is great with Jalapeño Spiced Coleslaw, found in the Sides section. Feel free to use any kind of white fish, although I prefer tilapia. Serve with a platter of accompaniments and let everyone build their own. Serve with Tomatillo Salsa found in the Appetizer section.

12 ounces tilapia or other flakey white fish
4 teaspoons grilling spice
8 10-inch flour tortillas
½ cup reduced-fat cheddar cheese
1 avocado

Grill the tilapia over medium heat until cooked through; depending on the thickness of the fish, 5 to 10 minutes. Remove fish from the grill. Place the tortillas on the grill and heat for a minute or so on each side. Place fish, cheese and avocado into tortillas to make a taco. Optionally, serve tortillas and fish on a large platter with sauces and sides for build-your-own fish tacos. Suggested sides: reduced-fat cheddar cheese, avocado or guacamole, Tomatillo Salsa, Jalapeño Spiced Coleslaw, jalapeño slices.

| Calories 224 | Fat 8.6g | Protein 18.8g | Carbs 18.9g | Sodium 544mg | Sugar 0.0 | Fiber 1.63g |

Seafood Cioppino   Serves 12

We love this stew after a day on the slopes or at the end of a cold winter day. Fast and easy to prepare, this stew is elegant enough for guests. Serve with a loaf of crusty bread to soak up all the yummy goodness.

1 onion, chopped

3 cloves garlic, minced

4 cans tomato sauce, 14.5 ounce

1 can tomato paste, 6 ounce

2 cans Italian-style diced tomatoes

1 pound mussels

½ pound shrimp

½ pound tilapia or any white fish

½ pound scallops

2 teaspoons Trader Joe's Everyday Seasoning - optional

2 teaspoons Italian seasoning

2 teaspoons Herbs de Provence

Splash of red wine, optional

Red pepper flakes to taste, optional

Salt and pepper to taste

Sauté the garlic and onion until soft and translucent; do not brown. Add the tomato sauce, paste and diced tomatoes to a large soup or stew pot. Add the Everyday Seasoning, Italian seasoning, Herbs de Provence and red pepper flakes to taste. Bring to a boil, reduce heat and simmer 20 minutes. Add the mussels, cook 3 minutes then add the remainder of the fish. Add a splash of red wine if desired. Cook 10 to 15 minutes until fish is cooked through. Add salt and pepper to taste. Serve.

Calories 79	Fat 0.97g	Protein 8.32g	Carbs 7.6g	Sodium 552mg	Sugar 1.6	Fiber 0.33g

Middle Eastern Chicken with Dried Fruit

Serves 4

A mix of Middle Eastern spices, dried fruit and olives add an exotic taste to this chicken dish. The chicken is moist and tender, with a sweet and savory mix of flavors. This is great over brown rice, quinoa or couscous.

1 teaspoon olive oil
4 garlic cloves, minced
1 teaspoon fresh ginger, minced
1 teaspoon ground cumin
½ teaspoon paprika
¼ teaspoon turmeric
¼ teaspoon cinnamon
¼ teaspoon salt

¼ teaspoon pepper
1 pound boneless chicken thighs
¼ cup chicken broth
¼ cup dried apricots, chopped
2 pitted dates, chopped
10 kalamata olives, pitted and
   chopped
1 tablespoon lemon zest, grated

Place the chicken thighs in a large zip-lock plastic bag. Combine the oil, garlic, ginger, cumin, paprika, turmeric, cinnamon, salt and pepper. Add to chicken, seal and shake to cover chicken. Refrigerate 3 hours or preferably overnight, turning occasionally. Spray a large nonstick pan with cooking spray. Add the chicken and the broth; set leftover marinade aside. Cook covered about 15 minutes. Turn chicken, add the apricots, dates, olives, lemon zest and 2 tablespoons of the marinade. Cook covered for an additional 15 minutes or until chicken is cooked through. If liquid cooks off, add 1 or 2 tablespoons of the reserved marinade or water.

Calories 200	Fat 6.6g	Protein 26.6g	Carbs 13.0g	Sodium 469mg	Sugar 7.1	Fiber 01.25g

SIDE DISHES

Quinoa with Herbs   Serves 6

6 cups chicken broth
½ cup lemon juice
3 cups quinoa
For dressing:
6 tablespoons lemon juice
3 tablespoons olive oil
¾ cup fresh basil, chopped
½ cup fresh flat leaf parsley, chopped
2 tablespoons fresh thyme, chopped
4 teaspoons lemon zest
Salt and pepper to taste

Bring broth to a boil in a medium saucepan. Add ½ cup lemon juice and quinoa. Return to a boil, reduce heat and simmer for 15 minutes or until liquid has absorbed and quinoa is tender. To make the dressing, add 6 tablespoons lemon juice, herbs, olive oil, and lemon zest together; mix thoroughly. Season to taste with salt and pepper. Toss dressing with quinoa and serve.

Calories 287	Fat 7.0g	Protein 11.0g	Carbs 44.0g	Sodium 47mg	Sugar 4.5	Fiber 5.0g

Jalapeño Spiced Coleslaw   Serves 6

This is definitely not you're mother's coleslaw. Light and refreshing, it packs a kick from the jalapeños. Make it as mild or hot as you like.

½ cup Fage non-fat yogurt
½ reduced-fat mayonnaise
¼ cup fresh cilantro, chopped
2 tablespoons rice wine vinegar
2 teaspoons sugar
½ teaspoon salt
½ teaspoon pepper
1 bag pre-shredded coleslaw
1 onion, chopped
10 jalapeño slices, chopped

In a small bowl, combine the yogurt, mayonnaise, vinegar, sugar, salt and pepper. Add the cilantro to the yogurt mixture. In a large bowl, combine the coleslaw, onion and jalapeño peppers; toss. Add the dressing and toss until well mixed. Refrigerate until ready to serve. For added color and crunch: add shredded carrots, red cabbage, sliced red pepper, jicama or sliced water chestnuts.

| Calories 63 | Fat 2.7g | Protein 2.4g | Carbs 7.9g | Sodium 183mg | Sugar 5.7 | Fiber 1.3g |

Sweet Potato Rounds   Serves 4

These tasty treats are so good they could almost be considered dessert! Crunchy on the outside, soft and sweet on the inside, you'll find you can't eat just a few.

3 large sweet potatoes
3 tablespoons olive oil
Sea salt and pepper to taste

Slice the potatoes into rounds, about ¼ inch thick. Toss with olive oil, salt and pepper in a large bowl. Spread onto a rimmed baking sheet. Cook in a preheated oven at 350 degrees for 12 minutes. Turn and cook for an additional 12 minutes or until golden brown.

Calories 191	Fat 10.4g	Protein 1.6g	Carbs 23.7g	Sodium 37mg	Sugar 0.0	Fiber 0.0g

Veggie Stir Fry with Spaghetti Squash   Serves 8

Using spaghetti squash instead of pasta noodles makes this stir-fry light, delicious and good for you.

1 spaghetti squash, about 3 pounds
1 medium red onion, chopped
3 cloves garlic, minced
2 carrots, julienned
2 red bell peppers, seeded and julienned
2 yellow bell peppers, seeded and julienned
1 cup broccoli florets
3 large tomatoes, seeded and chopped
1 cup chicken broth
¼ cup fresh basil, chopped
½ cup grated Parmesan cheese

Preheat the oven to 350 degrees. Cut the spaghetti squash in half lengthwise, scoop out the seeds and spray with cooking spray. Place cut side up on a rimmed baking sheet and cook for 30 minutes or until soft when pierced with a fork. Allow to cool slightly and then use a fork to scoop out the pulp. Spray a very large skillet or wok with cooking spray and heat on medium high. Add the onion, garlic, carrots, bell pepper and broccoli. Cook until tender-crisp, about 8 minutes. Stir in squash, broth, tomatoes and basil and heat through. Add the Parmesan cheese and toss. Season to taste with salt and pepper.

Calories 82	Fat 2.4g	Protein 3.9g	Carbs 10.6g	Sodium 127mg	Sugar 1.6	Fiber 53.5g

Spicy Black Bean Salad   Serves 4

This refreshing black bean salad comes with a kick. I prefer to use sliced jalapeños that come in a jar because they are easy to chop and I always have them available. Use fresh jalapeños if you prefer but reduce the amount as they tend to be hotter than those in a jar.

1 can black beans, 14.5 ounce, rinsed and drained
½ avocado, chopped
¼ cup cilantro
1 scallion, chopped
½ can of corn, 14.5 ounce
1 red bell pepper, chopped
4 tablespoons sliced jalapeños, chopped
2 tablespoons lime juice
1 tablespoon olive oil
Salt and pepper to taste

In a medium bowl, combine the beans, avocado, cilantro, scallions, jalapeño, lime juice and olive oil. Serve.

| Calories 178 | Fat 9.6g | Protein 5.3g | Carbs 19.5g | Sodium 101mg | Sugar 0.3 | Fiber 3.1g |

APPETIZERS

Cherry Tomato Poppers   Serves 8

This quick and easy appetizer is simple to make and tastes delicious. Use homegrown tomatoes or tomatoes from your local farmers market. Try popping them in the oven for a few minutes; they taste just as good warm.

32 cherry tomatoes
16 sliced jalapeños
4 low-fat mozzarella sticks or string cheese sticks

Slice off the top of the cherry tomatoes; spoon out insides. Place ½ of a jalapeño slice and a ½-inch slice of the string cheese or mozzarella stick inside each tomato. Serve cold or bake for 5 minutes before serving.

Calories 48	Fat 2.5g	Protein 4.2g	Carbs 2.2g	Sodium 205mg	Sugar 0.9	Fiber 0.4g

Black Bean Dip with Tortilla Triangles   Serves 8

This dip is simple and easy to whip up if guests arrive unexpectedly. Add a side of salsa and guacamole and you've got yourself a party. For a low carb treat, serve it with sliced jicama, carrots or other vegetables.

You'll probably use canned or bottled salsa in this recipe, but for the best homemade salsa ever, look for H & H Brand 30-second salsa. Just add petite diced tomatoes, let it sit for an hour and serve. 1 can makes 24 15-ounce servings. You can find it online at www.hnhbrands.com

1 can black beans, rinsed and
    drained
1 cup cilantro, chopped
½ cup salsa
½ cup fat free yogurt or fat free
    sour cream

1 teaspoon cumin
¼ teaspoon salt
¼ teaspoon pepper
2 tablespoons diced green chilies,
    optional

Place beans in a food processor with the cilantro, salsa, yogurt, cumin, salt and pepper. Blend. If using green chilies, add and serve.

You can also serve this dip hot. Place in ovenproof dish; sprinkle your choice of cheese on top. (I like cheddar or pepper jack, but any cheese will do). Cover with foil and bake in a 350 degree oven for 15 - 20 minutes or until heated through. Remove foil and bake an additional 5 to 10 minutes until cheese is melted and bubbly. Serve.

This recipe calls for flour tortillas, but feel free to substitute corn, whole wheat or flavored tortillas.

8 flour tortillas, 6 inch
Cooking spray
Sea salt to taste

Cut each tortilla into 8 triangles. Spray lightly with cooking spray and sprinkle with salt. Place on a rimmed baking sheet. Place in a 350 degree oven and bake for 5 to 7 minutes until just starting to brown. Turn tortilla chips over and bake an additional 5 minutes until golden brown. Serve.

| Calories 85 | Fat 1.3g | Protein 4.2g | Carbs 12.9g | Sodium 216mg | Sugar 0.9 | Fiber 0.7g |

White Bean and Sun-Dried Tomato Dip   Serves 8

This dip tastes great with a vegetable platter, crackers or Tortilla Triangles (see Black Bean Dip with Tortilla Triangles in the Appetizer section).

1 can white beans, drained and rinsed

2 tablespoons sundried tomatoes, chopped

2 tablespoons fresh basil,

1 tablespoon olive oil

Pinch of salt

2 cloves garlic, minced

1 scallion, chopped

½ cup non-fat sour cream

¼ cup pine nuts

Place beans, tomatoes, basil, olive oil garlic and scallion in a food processor. Blend until just combined, but you can still see bits of the vegetables. Stir in the sour cream. Transfer to serving bowl, cover and refrigerate for at least an hour. Sprinkle with pine nuts and slivers of basil leaves. Serve.

Calories 94	Fat 5.6g	Protein 3.7g	Carbs 10.0g	Sodium 133mg	Sugar 1.3	Fiber 1.7g

Tomatillo Salsa   Serves 8

Great with chips or with our Fish Tacos (see the recipe in the Dinner section).

20 tomatillos, husked and rinsed
1 medium onion, sliced
4 garlic cloves, unpeeled
1 chipotle in adobo sauce
2 tablespoons cilantro
Pinch of salt and sugar to taste

Broil the tomatillos, onion and garlic until charred. Peel the garlic and puree in a food processor with the tomatillos, onion, chipotle, cilantro. Add a pinch of salt and sugar to taste. Serve.

Calories 41	Fat 0.9g	Protein 1.1g	Carbs 44.0g	Sodium 31mg	Sugar 4.4	Fiber 2.1g

Raita with Naan Bread   Serves 8

An Indian-inspired dish, our Raita features non-fat yogurt making it light and refreshing. Serve with Naan bread to cool down any spicy dish.

2 cups non-fat yogurt, preferably Fage brand
2 cucumbers, peeled, seeded, grated and squeezed dry
3 sliced jalapeños, chopped
2 tablespoons fresh mint, chopped
1 teaspoon cumin
¼ teaspoon coriander
¾ teaspoon salt

If you are using Fage Greek yogurt there is no need to drain the yogurt. If using traditional yogurt, place the yogurt in a cheesecloth-lined strainer over a bowl and let drain for 30 minutes. Discard the liquid. In a bowl, combine the yogurt, cucumbers, jalapeño, mint, cumin, coriander and salt. Serve with Naan bread.

1 package Naan bread
Note: Naan can be found in most grocery stores and Trader Joe's.

Calories 80	Fat 2.1g	Protein 3.5g	Carbs 10.5g	Sodium 15mg	Sugar 1.8	Fiber 0.6g

Special Bonus Offer

Claim your free bonuses today!

Are you ready to start now to change your level of health and fitness?

Get $677 worth of free strategies, tips and tools to get you started right away.

Resources you will receive include:

- Online book exercises
- Fitness Assessment
- Great foods for travel
- Pack right for travel video
- Travel workout program
- And more....

To claim your free bonuses – visit us at:

www.slimpreneur.com/bookbonus

Enter your name and email and we'll send you a link to our members only resource area where you'll get all the free resources listed above and more. We're constantly adding and updating our valuable strategies, tips and tools so come back often and see what's new!

And REMEMBER – tell a friend about this book!

People always remember the person who first turned them on to new strategies that change their lives.

Be that person.